FROM INVISIBLE TO INVINCIBLE

THE NATURAL MENOPAUSE REVOLUTION

FROM INVISIBLE TO INVINCIBLE

THE NATURAL MENOPAUSE REVOLUTION

JENNIFER HARRINGTON, N.D.

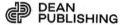

DEAN PUBLISHING

First published in 2020 by Dean Publishing
PO Box 119
Mt. Macedon, Victoria, 3441
Australia
deanpublishing.com

Cataloguing-in-Publication Data
National Library of Australia
Title: From Invisible To Invincible – The Natural Menopause Revolution
Edition: 1st edn
ISBN: 978-1-925452-22-8
Category: Women's Health

The views and opinions expressed in this book are those of the author
and do not necessarily reflect the official policy or position of any other
agency, publisher, organization, employer or company. Assumptions
made in the analysis are not reflective of the position of any entity other
than the author(s) — and, these views are always subject to change,
revision, and rethinking at any time.

The author, publisher or organizations are not to be held responsible for
misuse, reuse, recycled and cited and/or uncited copies of content within
this book by others.

This book is not intended as a substitute for the medical advice of
physicians. The reader should regularly consult a physician in matters
relating to his/her health and particularly with respect to any symptoms
that may require diagnosis or medical attention. The ideas within this
book are only the the opinion of the author and are not intended to
replace any medical advice or health issues.

This book is dedicated to my amazing daughter Emily.

You are my sunshine.

Jennifer is sharing more in her INTERACTIVE book.

See exclusive, behind-the-scenes videos, audios and photos.

DOWNLOAD free content and go *From Invisible To Invincible*.

deanpublishing.com/invincible

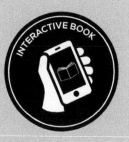

CONTENTS

it's not about your hormones

"If menopause symptoms were due solely to hormonal changes then the menopausal experience would be more homogenous."
— *Dr Sandra Thompson,*
University of Western Australia

That's right ladies. Stop blaming your hormones.

The fact is, every woman will stop menstruating at some point. The natural production of estrogen, progesterone, and testosterone will reduce, but not all women will suffer during this transition. If lower hormones were the problem, all women would suffer equally. The hormones load the gun, but what pulls the trigger?

It's what you have done over your lifetime that will determine the severity of your symptoms.

This acts as a trigger for the metaphorical gun. So, ask yourself:

- Have you lived a highly stressful life?
- Do you live on fast foods, consume too much alcohol or smoke?
- Have you been exposed to toxic substances like metals or chemicals or been exposed to excessive radiation?
- Are you living a sedentary lifestyle?
- Do you have any lingering infections? Certain viruses can stay in your body for life and can flare up from time to time causing unexplained symptoms.

Before you run away, let me tell you the great news. This can be changed. How? Stay tuned and I will explain. The best place to begin is with a definition.

Menopause is classified as the end of your periods, officially 12 months since your last period.

The average age for women in Australia is 51 years. The period after this age is defined as post-menopause. Post menopause is *not* a time of no reproductive hormones; it's a time of reduced hormone production. Other parts of your body will help to pick up the slack but not take over its production.

The adrenal gland is responsible for producing most of the reproductive hormones in menopause, but estrogen can also be metabolised by your adipose tissue (fat cells). This may be the reason why many women naturally gain a little weight in perimenopause, as this will help them produce estrogen after their ovaries have stopped producing.

Perimenopause is the transitional phase that happens before menopause.

It can start as early as 10 years before menopause. Women as early as mid-thirties can start to feel the change in their hormonal status. In the early stages, your ovaries reduce the frequency of ovulation. You may still menstruate, but the frequency, duration, and quantity of blood can change. If you didn't ovulate this month, your production of progesterone in the second half of your cycle would be negligible. Your estrogen levels might not change, but the ratio between the amount of estrogen you have, compared to the amount of progesterone you have, is imbalanced. This is referred to as having relative estrogen dominance. Early signs of this include anxiety and sleep alterations.

If you reach menopause before the age of 40 regardless of whether it was natural or due to surgery or chemotherapy, this is called premature menopause. For a small number of women, this can come tragically too soon and rob them of their fertile years. For these women, this book cannot help restore their fertility, but it can help reduce their symptoms and help them manage long-term conditions associated with low hormones such as osteoporosis.

On the other hand, women going through perimenopause make up the second largest group of women having babies. Please note, irregular periods do not equal infertility. It is important to maintain contraception during this time if you do not wish to expand your family.

It is also a time of increased sexually transmitted infections. If you are re-entering the singles scene or have multiple sexual partners, please refresh your memory about safe sex and condoms. Have fun, but play safe. Don't become part of the statistics.

– – –

Most women will experience natural menopause—the slow reduction of hormones over time—with or without symptoms. Other women are thrust headfirst into an overnight menopausal state as a result of surgery or chemotherapy. Unfortunately, this can cause a more intense start to their symptoms. Luckily, I have successfully used these same natural strategies to help resolve symptoms for these women. But again, the severity of symptoms experienced can be related to their lifestyle. Lots of stress and burnt out adrenals aren't going to do you any favours.

For the sake of convenience during this book when I refer to 'menopausal symptoms', I am talking about perimenopausal and menopausal symptoms together. That being, the process or transition from being fertile to infertile.

THE TRANSITORY PHASE: FROM WE TO ME

The transitory phase of moving from fertile to infertile is often overlooked in society, however it's a very powerful time if understood. It is often explained as a transition from *we* to *me*. Transition from thinking about life as a group, to life as an individual. From the primary focus being your partner, kids, extended family and community, to thinking about yourself. Due to this significant change in life-view, it can be a time of extreme turmoil. The highest amounts of divorce happen during this transition. This demographic is also the most likely to quit their job and venture into the world as self-employed new business owners. Go, girl! It's very much a time where you stop taking crap from anyone dishing it out (e.g., ex-husbands, old bosses and old friends). You no longer accept being pushed around full stop. Most women find themselves speaking their minds—sometimes to their own surprise.

It is also a time for self-reflection and growth. A time to re-establish your identity. Many women contemplate their existence and look for more meaning in life, especially in relation to the broader community. Asking questions like: How do I contribute to society? Should I volunteer or fundraise? How do I make my life more meaningful?

Think of yourself as the caterpillar in your cocoon, battering your wings against the wall. It can be a tough time, but it doesn't last forever. Soon you will morph into a beautiful butterfly with new wings and a new world to explore. This book is designed to help strengthen your wings and get you out of your cocoon earlier. It is designed to help you explore your new life—symptom-free—with more confidence and renewed ideas of how to contribute fully to life, *starting with yours.*

Menopause and perimenopause needn't be a time of hell, so to speak. My goal for you is to achieve a shift in your symptoms and go forward in life with more satisfaction: better health, happier moods, closer bonds with family and friends and improved sex life. I want you to live the best life possible for you.

Throughout the book you will notice the Wonder Woman image. The Wonder Woman power pose, if held for two minutes, has been shown to increase testosterone levels, reduce cortisol, improve the ability to handle stress, increase pain tolerance and help induce abstract thinking. Add it to your morning routine before you leave the house each morning or do it in the bathroom before a big meeting.

Are you ready to get started?

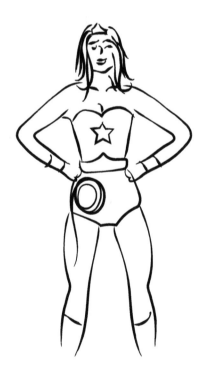

why western women suffer the most

It's fascinating to look at how women from different cultures and races view menopause. All women go through this change. For some women it's a time of dread, while for others it's a time to look forward to.

Your thoughts regarding this time of life can change your reality.

If you put energy into thinking something is wrong, it will most likely be bad. For many women, menopause is a time of celebration, a step-up the cultural ladder, a transition into being a wise woman. For others, it's the beginning of the end; a downward spiral into insignificance and death. Choose your thoughts wisely.

DIFFERENT WAYS OTHER CULTURES VIEW MENOPAUSE

Different cultures across the world view menopause differently. Not just the process, per se, but the very definition. In fact, some research has highlighted the complicated nature of menopausal studies due to differences between cultures—more specifically regarding the definition of menopause, reproductive histories, expression of symptoms and even beliefs within a society.

It's useful to highlight because it will help you recognise that across the world, our views, experiences and symptoms, may be different. While this period of our lives is inevitable, it's important to respect each other as women; and that our culture, our histories, our beliefs and our symptoms are what make this period of our lives sacred for each of us.

Let's look at some examples:
- Aboriginal women look forward to menopause. For these women, it is a 'step-up' in society; a time of improved status and an opportunity to become a leader in their clan.
- Mayan (Mexican) women also look forward to increased freedom and improved status. These women have slightly earlier menopause, are relatively symptom-free and enjoy an improved sex life afterwards!
- Papago (Native Americans) don't have a word for menopause. Perhaps the absence of a definition means this period of life assumes a more natural symptom-free approach?
- In Japan, the main symptom of menopause is a stiff shoulder, followed by headaches and muscle pain. Interestingly there isn't a word in the Japanese language for hot flushes. The closest word in Japanese for the translation for menopause is 'Konenki', which is used to describe a positive transitional stage in life.

- Women from Hong Kong report similar issues as the Japanese, with muscle pain and joint problems as initial symptoms.
- Nigerian women also complain about muscle pain, but not hot flushes.
- Filipino women struggle with headaches.
- Lebanese women's biggest complaint is fatigue and mood swings.
- Indian women appear to experience little symptoms. This was demonstrated in a study of 483 Indian women who had stopped menstruating. These women did however experience positive social changes, including the opportunity to socialise with men, joke and drink homebrew.
- In Northern Thailand, the Meo tribe have a celebratory ritual to mark menopause.
- Pagan's see this stage of life as the 'crone'; a time for visibility, acceptance and celebration. It is a time to look forward to and considered a passageway to becoming the much anticipated 'elder woman'. The elder women roles have a responsibility to be role models to other women. It is considered an honour and an achievement.
- Chinese call menopause 'the second spring' and view it as a positive stage of life.
- Across the world, there are also various rituals and ceremonies. For example, there is a modern-day ritual called 'The Woman's 14th Moon Ceremony',[1] that celebrates a woman on her '14th moon'. This means that the woman has gone through 13 full moons in one year without menstruating and is celebrated as an elder and wise woman.

---

1. Women of the 14th Moon, 2016. http://www.womenofthe14thmoon.com

The post-menopausal decades should be golden years to look forward to and enjoy. After all, the Chinese believe life begins at 60!

Western society needs to start changing our views on older women. We need to collectively stop devaluing older women and worshipping youth. Instead, it's time to celebrate the ageing process and the new freedom this stage allows. After all, it wasn't always like this. Societal views on older women were not always perceived as negative. Take for example the use of words and how they have changed in meaning over time. Have you ever heard an older woman being called a 'hag'? In today's society, being called a 'hag' is derogative. It conjures up images of evil, vicious, malicious and ugly. However, the term 'hag' used to be a positive word, meaning wise woman, teacher or fairy. In Irish and Scottish mythology, the 'hag' was a goddess linked with creations, harvest, weather and sovereignty. However, it's not just words that have changed over time, it's our perceived value. Just as we once relied on our wise women to lead to way, we now cut them down. This must stop. Our knowledge and experience are too valuable. This change needs to start with us, from us. When you look in the mirror who do you see? We can't expect the world to love us if we don't love and value ourselves.

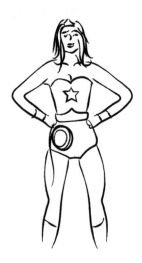

what's happening? why me?

I'm often asked why some women experience menopausal symptoms but not all. Good question.

The exact mechanism is unknown. What we do know however, is there is a part in your brain called the hypothalamus which is responsible for temperature regulation, sex drive, sleep, moods and memory. This area contains many estrogen receptors. Estrogen is needed to bind to these receptors for the hypothalamus to work effectively. When estrogen levels start to drop, this causes changes in the way the hypothalamus functions and as such, symptoms may occur.

However, the issue can be two-fold. It can be the reduction of available estrogen to bind to the receptors, or it can be that the receptors are 'dirty' or dysfunctional. They may be clogged and unable to accept any available estrogen. Receptors become dirty when exposed to xenoestrogens, toxic metals and other toxic chemicals. Please read the section on *Non-toxic environment* to learn more. Healthy receptors need available co-factors for optimal functioning. Co-factors are nutrients that encourage and allow hormones to bind. These include important nutrients such as zinc, B vitamins, iodine, vitamin A and magnesium.

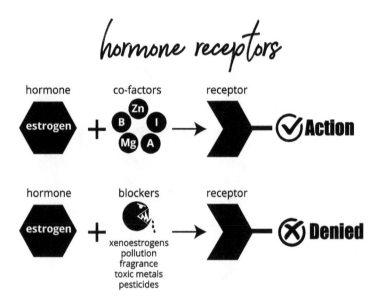

Estrogen receptors are not just found in the reproductive system and brain; they are also in your skin, breast tissue, adrenals, bladder, kidney, bone, joints, lung, intestines, thymus, lymphatic vessels, heart and blood vessels. Wherever the receptors are located, we can experience changes in function once the available estrogen levels have reduced or the receptors have become dysfunctional.

estrogen receptors

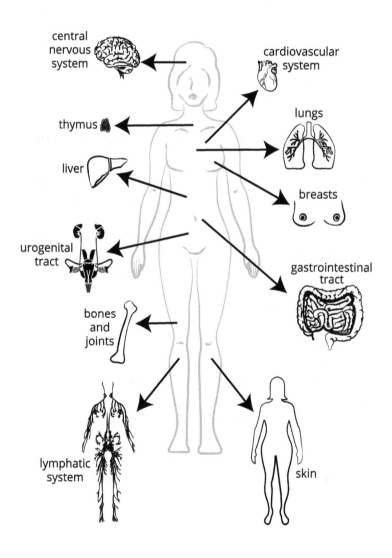

In your reproductive years, your ovaries produce estrogen, but as your ovaries start to fail and your levels reduce, they send a feedback loop to your brain to produce even more ovarian stimulants: follicle stimulating hormone (FSH) and luteinising hormone (LH). If you took a blood test during this time, you would see high levels of FSH and LH. I view these elevated hormones as your brains way of screaming at your ovaries to function. The more exhausted your ovaries are, the more FSH and LH the brain produces—but it's the beginning of the end for your ovaries. Your ovaries will continue to produce small amounts of hormones, but it's at this stage it recruits the adrenal glands to help.

HOW DOES YOUR LIFESTYLE AFFECT YOUR SYMPTOMS?

If you have ever seen me speak publicly, you would have undoubtedly heard me emphasise the importance of adrenal health.

One of the biggest differences between women who have symptoms and those who don't can be directly related to the amount of long-term stress they have experienced over their lifetime.

This is a MAJOR concern as I don't know anyone who lives stress-free their entire life. Some stress can be beneficial, such as an assignment deadline, but long-term multi-factorial stress is a massive issue. Many women have raised kids, looked after the household, held down a full-time job. Some remain carers for their parents or have the added burden of financial stress. *It's not one stressful experience, it's many.*

Your adrenal glands produce your stress hormones— adrenaline, noradrenalin, cortisol, and DHEA. If your adrenal glands are stimulated too hard and for too long, you still start experiencing adrenal dysfunction.

Adrenal dysfunction and stress

Adrenal dysfunction produces very similar symptoms to menopause: night sweats, fatigue, muscular aches, headaches, brain fog and mood issues such as anxiety and depression. It's hard to tell what is coming from your adrenals and what is from your lack of reproductive hormones. The adrenals also take over the production of your hormones once your ovaries start to shut down. The adrenal glands already have a full work schedule and if you overload them, don't expect a good production of reproductive hormones later. If this sounds like you (let me tell you, it sounds like me) don't worry, all hope is not lost. We will go over strategies to improve adrenal function later.

But for now, start thinking about where your stress is coming from and how you can turn that around. Removal of the stressful situation is ideal but not always possible, e.g., a sick relative. Throughout the book, we will discuss techniques such as exercise and meditation to help manage your stress levels and supplements such as magnesium to help optimise function.

Liver function and toxic load

Your liver is responsible for keeping your body clean. It detoxifies and removes dangerous substances from your body. It also produces and regulates hormones. If your liver is overwhelmed and overworked, it will try to prioritise cleaning the body and keeping you alive and therefore, won't be able to regulate your hormone levels successfully. Your liver function will also be reduced if it's fatty. Fatty liver can be alcohol or dietary (carbohydrate) related. It's essential to help promote optimal liver function at all stages of life, but especially during menopause.

What is even scarier is that the hypothalamus, pituitary and pineal gland (sections of the brain that regulate hormones and sleep) are not protected by the blood-brain barrier.

What this means is that toxins have direct access to these particular parts of the brain, and they can be stored there.

These toxins have an affinity for the brain: mercury, lead, aluminium, PCB, solvents, and dioxins. They can cause symptoms such as hormonal imbalance, brain fog, insomnia, memory issues, fatigue, headache, depression, anxiety and more. It's important to investigate for toxicity issues before starting hormonal treatment. Hormonal treatment may band-aid the symptoms while these toxins sit undiscovered, having longer to damage the brain. It's so important to investigate to make sure you find the true underlying cause and not temporarily prop yourself up for a temporary solution.

Now, before you protest and say, 'That's not me, I don't live in a toxic area, I have always eaten organic foods and used chemical-free products,' …well, I'm sorry to say that it may in fact be you. It's all of us to some degree. The Environmental Working Group (EWG) released a study called *10 Americans*[2] which investigated the umbilical cord blood of ten random babies. The study found that each baby contained on average, 200 different industrial pollutants and chemicals even before being born! We are living in a world of toxins, which is why it's so important to identify your toxin/s and detoxify them.

As suggested in the study you don't need to be exposed to toxins directly for them to affect you. Researchers have found toxic exposure doesn't just affect you, it can affect multiple future generations as well. In fact, current research has indicated up to three generations, but as time goes on, this may be increased to more. Think about the industrial pollutants your parents or grandparents may have been exposed to and how they might still be affecting you.

In later chapters, you will find information about cleaning your home and removing toxic chemicals. The less chemicals you are exposed to, the less work your liver needs to do to

2. https://www.ewg.org/news/videos/10-americans

remove them—which means the liver can then focus on balancing or producing new hormones.

What you eat also impacts on your liver function. If you are eating the standard Australian or American diet (appropriately named The SAD diet[3]) this encourages both the development of fatty liver and increases the toxicity of the body due to the number of preservatives, colours, flavours, pesticides, etc. found in food. See the section on 'Nutritious foods' for more information on how to eat to promote better liver function and health in general.

If you have ever seen a naturopath, you would have heard us say, 'It all starts in the gut'. Menopause is no different. The digestive microbiome is responsible for synthesising and secreting hormones, regulating the expression of hormones, inhibiting the production of some hormones and enhancing the production of others. So, if your digestive system works well, your hormones are generally balanced. If your digestive system isn't what it used to be, your hormones could be all over the place. The subset of the digestive microbiome that is responsible for metabolising estrogen is called the estrobolome. A healthy estrobolome balances estrogen levels by excreting excess, but if the estrobolome is imbalanced beta-glucuronidase is produced—an enzyme that can prevent estrogen clearance and promote estrogen excess.

Viral infections

The herpes family of viruses is larger than you probably realise and effects about 95 percent of the population. HSV 1 is the common cold sore while HSV 2 is the genital variety (although this can also be the other way around). Other members of the family include epstein barr virus (glandular fever), cytomegalovirus

---

3. The standard American diet (SAD), is known in wider circles for its excess sugar, refined carbohydrates, saturated fat and trans fats. It is the primary cause of obesity and diabetes. Although the SAD diet was named after the American style of eating, this eating pattern has spread around the world contributing to obesity and health issues.

(glandular fever), varicocella zoster (chicken pox, shingles) human herpes 6 (roseola), human herpes 7 (roseola) and human herpes 8 (kaposi's sarcoma). Once infected, the herpes virus stays with you and may become reactive intermittently. Some women experience viral flares and mistake this for their menopausal transition. Epstein barr virus is thought to be the most problematic strain. Chronic viral flares can cause fatigue, achy joints, night sweats, headaches, digestive issues, behavioural changes, depressive mood changes, nerve pain, tingling, rashes, itch, burning sensations and increased risk of cancer development. In this case you are better to work on reducing your viral load, rather than playing around with your hormones.

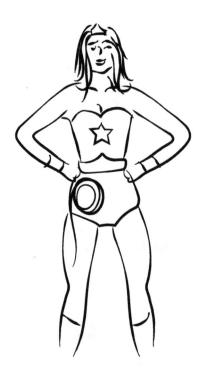

QUIZ TIME

How Many Symptoms Do You Have?

The first step of any journey is to acknowledge your beginning point.

Head over to the online Menopause Quiz, to get a good idea of how many menopause-related symptoms you have.

Once you begin implementing changes to your diet and lifestyle or start taking supplements, head back over and repeat the quiz.

It's a great way to monitor your improvements and see which changes had the most significant impact.

menopausenaturalsolutions.com/menopause-symptom-tracker-quiz

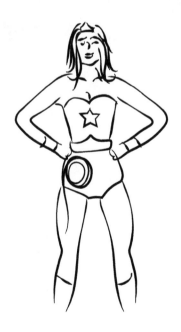

Jennifer is sharing more in her INTERACTIVE book.

See exclusive, behind-the-scenes videos, audios and photos.

DOWNLOAD free content and go *From Invisible To Invincible.*

deanpublishing.com/invincible

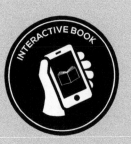

10 steps to becoming invincible

I often consult with women who are using hormone replacement and experiencing a lot of side-effects. When I ask them about their history, they all seem to have jumped from merely having symptoms to going straight on several medications. They started their journey with the final options instead of looking at alternatives in the beginning. I believe there is a time and place for everything. Some women do better on medication, but many women don't need anything this extreme.

I recommend women begin with the INVINCIBLE strategy first, then see if any symptoms remain before starting specific treatment. If you're already on medication, you can use the INVINCIBLE method first and then discuss weaning off medication with your prescribing doctor later.

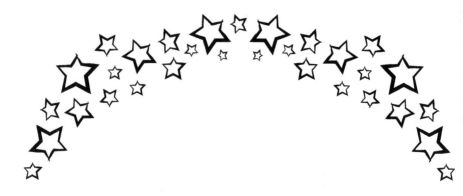

I	INDIVIDUALISED TREATMENT PLAN
N	NUTRITIOUS FOODS
V	VITAMINS AND MINERALS
I	INVESTIGATE
N	NON-TOXIC ENVIRONMENT
C	CONTRIBUTION
I	INTUITION
B	BREATHE
L	LOVE YOUR LIVER AND DETOX
E	EXERCISE AND OTHER LIFESTYLE FACTORS

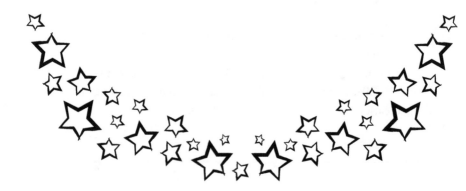

i = individual treatment plan

You are a unique woman! There is no one else on the planet like you. Therefore, it makes sense that your road to wellness will be equally unique. Many deficiencies are common, and often I recommend similar solutions, but the form of the nutrient or the dose or duration, may be very different from one woman to the next.

No two women have the same needs. Please don't start a one-size-fits-all approach to your health. You deserve better.

n = nutritious foods

"Let food be thy medicine"
— Hippocrates

What should we be eating? There are few subjects as confusing as nutrition. Countless diets exist on the market, all contradicting each other. One claims to eat this, the next to avoid that. It's no wonder people are confused! It's time to get back to basics.

We should be eating how Mother Nature intended us to. She provides us with countless variety of foods, yet we mostly eat 'food-like' substances manufactured in a laboratory. Do you remember eating at your grandparents' house? I can guarantee they were eating more homemade meals with food straight from the farm. The meals themselves would have had only a few ingredients.

Have you heard of the Farm to Fork initiative?[4] This initiative encourages you to eat mostly locally grown, freshly farmed

4. Farm to Fork Initiative, 2019. https://www.farmtoforkinitiative.org

produce that hasn't used life-extending chemicals on the food, as it won't have been transported long distances or stored for long periods of time. This way of eating encourages you to eat seasonally. It also increases the nutrition of the food, as fruits and vegetables that need to be transported are often picked unripe and artificially ripened after long storage periods. This also reduces the carbon footprint of the food, making it better for the planet. The ultimate Farm to Fork idea is to grow produce yourself—however it's unlikely you will produce everything you need. I grow some food and buy the rest at my local farmers market. I love that it puts money directly into the farmers hand rather than diluting their income by shopping through supermarkets. If you can't make the day of the market, there are a lot of online shops that will deliver a box of fresh local produce to your door. An added benefit on the Farm to Fork initiative is getting to know your farmer. I get so much inspiration from the farmers at my local market; they love a good yarn and often give me tips for my own garden and recipes. One of the farmers at my local market allows camping on their farm; a real farm-stay experience.

If you live in Australia, I encourage you to find your local farmers market and go shopping. The Australian Farmers Market Association directory is a useful tool:

farmersmarkets.org.au/find-a-market

How to know good food when you see it

You should be able to identify your food. For example, a cob of corn is easily identified as corn, but can you say the same for corn chips? No! The only way you know corn is inside is by the name, but it appears nothing like the original food. Most retail corn chips contain more than 20 other ingredients. As a rule, the more processed the food, the larger the number of ingredients on the label.

GENETICALLY MODIFIED FOOD

Genetically modified (GM) food is food that has had its DNA changed in order to create a more desirable outcome for the farmer. For example, growing a crop that is resistant to the herbicide glycosate (Roundup) so it can be sprayed to kill bugs without killing the plant. Did you know this isn't just happening with crops, there are also genetically modified animals such as salmon?

The truth is, we don't know the effects of genetically modified food—nor will we know for several decades. I don't want to be a guinea pig and I don't want you to be either. Australia and the US are very open to GM foods. In other parts of the world, these foods are banned or strictly restricted. Please consider for a moment how you feel about GM foods, considering some countries don't consider these safe.

Countries with GM prohibitions:
- Algeria
- Austria
- Azerbaijan
- Belize
- Bhutan
- Bosnia and Herzegovina
- Bulgaria
- Croatia
- Cyprus
- Denmark
- Ecuador
- France
- Germany
- Greece
- Hungary
- Italy
- Kenya
- Kyrgyzstan

- Latvia
- Lithuania
- Luxembourg
- Madagascar
- Malta
- Moldova
- Netherlands
- Northern Ireland, Scotland, Wales (United Kingdom)
- Norway
- Peru
- Poland
- Russia
- Saudi Arabia
- Serbia
- Slovenia
- Switzerland
- Turkey
- Ukraine
- Venezuela
- Zimbabwe.

The Genetic Literacy Project[5] provides a useful tool that answers many common facts and questions about GM foods.

In the meantime, avoiding GM foods is a wise choice—not only because they are modified but because these foods are generally highly sprayed foods. This means that no matter how well the food is washed before consuming, there will always be traces remaining in the food.

The following foods are highly modified and are best to avoid:
- Soy (94% is genetically modified)
- Corn (92% is genetically modified)
- Canola
- Cotton.

5. https://gmo.geneticliteracyproject.org/FAQ/where-are-gmos-grown-and-banned

Food for thought: even if the animal hasn't been genetically modified, it may have been fed GM foods. The effect of this is also unknown.

WHY EAT ORGANIC FOOD?

Organic food is GM free. It hasn't been sprayed with toxic, cancer forming herbicides and pesticides, such as glycosphate. This is the most common reason for eating organic food.

Organic foods are prohibited from using biosolids, a fancy name for sewage sludge. Conventional farming uses biosolids as fertilisers, however the problem is, this sewage waste can contain heavy metals and be contaminated with pathogens. Not something I want on my food.

Organic food does not use growth promoting drugs like ractopamine, which is banned in the European Union, Russia and China, but not Australia. Also, organic food does not use antibiotics.

Ideally you would eat as organically as you can afford. In a perfect world, it would be 100% organic, but this isn't cheap and not everything is available everywhere. As a starting point, I recommend you only eat these foods when they are organic. These foods have also been coined the Dirty Dozen[6]. They are the 12 most highly sprayed crops. Removing these foods from your diet will remove 80% of your pesticide load.[7] What a great way to start.

MOST TOXIC COMMERCIALLY GROWN FOOD
1. Strawberries
2. Spinach
3. Nectarines
4. Apples
5. Grapes

6. Environmental Working Group, 'Dirty Dozen' 2019. https://www.ewg.org/foodnews/dirty-dozen.php
7. ibid.

6. Peaches
7. Cherries
8. Pears
9. Tomato
10. Celery
11. Potato
12. Bell pepper/Capsicum.

If finances are tight, the following foods are the safest to eat in non-organic form. These foods have also been dubbed the Clean Fifteen.[8]

THE SAFEST NON-ORGANIC FOODS YOU CAN EAT ON A BUDGET

1. Avocado
2. Sweet corn (although low in pesticides, it is often genetically modified)
3. Pineapples
4. Cabbages
5. Onion
6. Sweet peas
7. Papaya/ pawpaw
8. Asparagus
9. Mangoes
10. Eggplant
11. Honeydew melon
12. Kiwi
13. Rockmelon
14. Cauliflower
15. Broccoli.

8. Environmental Working Group, 'Clean Fifteen' 2019. https://www.ewg.org/foodnews/clean-fifteen.php

MACRONUTRIENTS: THE MAIN BUILDING BLOCKS OF FOOD

There are three main components to food: carbohydrates, protein and fats.

CARBOHYDRATES

Carbohydrates are any food that can be broken down by the body into simple sugars.This includes fruit, vegetables, nuts, lentils, beans, grains, cereals, bread, rice, pasta, honey, sugar, soft drinks and baked goods such as muffins and cakes.

The amount of sugar hidden in each food type varies. Below are the average percentage amounts of sugar that your body converts each food type in to:

- Grains 75%
- Legumes 25%
- Nuts 20%
- Fruit 12%
- Vegetables 8%

Therefore, a normal serving of pasta (125 g) converts to around 94 g of sugar. Wow! That's a lot. To help you visual this amount, a teaspoon of sugar is 4 grams, so the amount of sugar your body converted your bowl of pasta into, is equivalent to eating 23.5 teaspoons of sugar. Let's hope you didn't include garlic bread and dessert and wash it down with a can of coke. That's a lot of sugar!

Sugar is used by the body as a fuel source, although the body can use other food sources for fuel (which is why they are called 'simple' sugars and not 'essential' sugars). Your body only uses sugar as an energy source. Too much of it causes weight gain, diabetes, fatigue, depletion of other nutrients, insomnia, acidity, reduced immunity, fatty liver, teeth cavities and weak bones. It also promotes heart disease, inflammation, causes brain fog, feeds cancer cells and is highly addictive.

Once the carbohydrates get broken down into sugar, a small part remains in the blood as an immediate fuel source. Next, a slightly larger amount is stored in your muscles and liver as glycogen. Glycogen is a short-term fuel supply that can easily be converted back to sugar if your body needs it. Finally, any leftover sugar is stored in the body as fat—a long-term fuel supply. As we rarely face famine these days, it's easy to start filling those fat stores and never burning them as fuel. Once they are laid down, they can't go back up the same metabolic pathway they came down. But it's not all bad news. A new direction is needed here. Fat can be redirected and broken down in the liver via the process of ketosis.

Considering carbohydrates break down to sugar, should we simply avoid all of them? No. Looking at the table above, fruit and vegetables average 10% sugar, which leaves 90% nutrition in the form of water, fibre, vitamins, minerals and phytonutrients. It's simply about looking at the type of carbohydrate you're consuming, rather than avoiding them altogether.

Tips for eating carbohydrates

- Vegetables and salads should be eaten in abundance. Anything grown above ground is generally lower in carbohydrates. Anything grown below ground, such as root vegetables like potatoes, are storehouses of sugar for the plant and are therefore higher in carbohydrates. Root vegetables are still ok to eat but most of your vegetables should be from above ground sources.
- The lowest carbohydrate fruits are berries and melons. Eat one to two serves of fruit every day.
- Nuts are a combination food, meaning they are a carbohydrate but also a protein and fat. My concern with nuts is mould. Any stored grain, seed or nut can be contaminated with mould. The best way to prevent this is to buy the freshest nuts possible and store them in the freezer instead of the cupboard. The healthiest nuts are activated nuts. You can buy these or make your own.

An important thing to remember about eating nuts is to eat a portion and not an entire bag.

- Consume legumes in moderation. Legumes are also a phytoestrogen, but more about that later.
- Grains are best to eat sparingly, if at all.
- Learn to identify and avoid other sources of sugars that are hidden in processed foods including white sugar, brown sugar, confectioners' sugar, corn syrup, dextrin, maltodextrin, honey, invert sugar, maple syrup, raw sugar, beet sugar, cane sugar, corn sweeteners, evaporated cane juice, high fructose corn syrup, malt, molasses, and anything ending in 'ose' (e.g., maltose, sucrose, lactose).

PROTEIN

Protein is broken down by the body into essential and non-essential amino acids. Essential means that you must consume this component as the human body cannot manufacture it. Therefore, eating foods that contain adequate amino acids is a must for a healthy and happy body.

Foods containing amino acids include:
- All animal products: meat, chicken, fish, eggs, dairy
- Vegetarian sources: nuts, seeds, lentils.

Amino acids are essential for:
- Every single cell in your body as they are a key building block for new cell creation.
- Building and repairing muscles, organs and other structural components of your body.
- Immune response (antibody formation).
- Energy (haemoglobin production—part of a red blood cell that carries oxygen).
- Building enzymes, neurotransmitters and hormones.
- Regulating body processes (e.g., water balance, transports nutrients).

Did you read the part about needing protein to form hormones? Some women find it a catch-22. They know they need to eat more protein, but unfortunately, they struggle to digest it, so avoid it. If this is you, you need more digestive fire, more enzymes and acids. Make sure you read the section on digestion.

Each meal you eat *must* contain some protein.

FATS

Did you know the body breaks down fats to form essential and non-essential fatty acids? Like protein, essential means that you must consume this macronutrient, as the human body cannot manufacture it. Therefore, eating fat-containing foods is a must.

Foods containing good fats include:
- Animal products: wild fish, organic eggs, kangaroo, grass-fed meats
- Vegetarian sources: olives, avocado, nuts, seeds, grasses, coconut.

Please do not consume low-fat products. Manufacturers have three main choices when it comes to flavouring foods: fat; sugar and salt. Fat is beneficial for human consumption; sugar and de-mineralised salt is harmful. As a golden rule for nutrition, look for the food which is least altered. It will be the best option every time.

Benefits
- Enables absorption and activation of fat-soluble nutrients (ADEK, calcium)
- Strengthens bones
- Increases sensation of fullness
- Production and regulation of hormones
- Nerve signalling, such as regulating insulin release
- Supports cellular structure and function (a key component of your cells phospholipid membrane)

- Reduces premature ageing
- Cancer preventing
- Muscle building
- Fat burning (*not* fat gaining)
- Provides energy
- Source of lubrication
- Anti-inflammatory
- Promotes hair, skin and nail health
- Supports brain health and cognitive function
- Promotes eye health
- Improves mood and behaviour
- Improves cardiovascular health
- Protects the liver from certain drugs and medications
- Encourages healthy lung function, as the lung coating surfactant is made from 100% fat
- Strengthens the immune system.

Types of Fat
Unsaturated fats
- Monounsaturated fats (olive, avocado, nuts, seeds)
- Polyunsaturated fats (fish, nuts, seeds, vegetable oil)
  - » Omega 3 (essential oil) (fish, grass)
    - EPA (arthritis, depression, inflammation, anticancer)
    - DHA (cardiovascular health and brain function)
  - » Omega 6 (palm, soybean, canola/rapeseed, sunflower, grains. The ideal ratio of Omega 6 to Omega 3 is 2:1. The typical Western diet is 30:1, which is too high, so best to avoid these sources)
  - » Omega 7 (sea buckthorn oil) (mucous membranes and skin health)
  - » Omega 9 (non-essential oil) (olives, avocado, nuts, seeds).

Saturated Fats
There is a common misconception that saturated fats are bad—however they are essential for health. Food sources include breast

milk, coconut, animal products, butter, bacon and cheese.

Benefits
- Enhances immunity
- Promotes heart health
- Helps build phospholipid membranes
- Prevents osteoporosis
- Helps reduce allergies.

Hydrogenated fats (supersaturated fats)
- CLA (natural fat found in sources such as kangaroo, meat, dairy, eggs). The benefits include decreasing body fat, increasing lean tissue, anti-cancer, heart health and decreasing inflammation.
- Trans fat (unhealthy, man-made fat found in fried foods, processed foods, baked foods, margarine).
- Interesterified fat (very unhealthy man-made hydrogenated 'trans-fat-free'. It's made so manufacturers can say they have a trans-fat-free product, but it's actually worse for you. It's not suitable for human consumption and is known to cause diabetes).

Please don't be afraid of adding the right kinds of fats into your diet. There have been decades of misinformation about dietary fats and I see people struggle with this information daily. The easy rule of thumb regarding fats is that naturally containing fats are beneficial for health while man-made fats or interfered with fats are very detrimental to health.

DRINKS

Consider the role of dehydration for a minute. A grape is well hydrated and looks plump, young and healthy, while a dehydrated raisin looks shrivelled up and old. The difference is water. How much are you drinking every day? The minimum you should be drinking is 2 litres. If you are not a water drinker, start with 1 litre and increase by 250 ml a week until you get there. If you increase too quickly, you will spend far too much time on the toilet. If you are still struggling, read the section on urinary frequency. Something that is far more important than the quantity of water you are drinking, is the quality of water. Please invest in a quality water filter.

Herbal teas can be very delicious and helpful during menopause. Sage is a traditional tea used to help reduce excessive sweat. It also has calming, anti-inflammatory and memory enhancing qualities. The tea can be drank with fresh or dried tea leaves. Fennel tea is usually considered a digestive drink, good for bloating, gas and cramps but it's also a good tea for menopause. It has been found to help reduce hot flushes and anxiety, while improving sleep.

Alcohol can trigger hot flushes in many women. Research on alcohol has found that moderate drinkers are less likely to develop dementia and more likely to live a longer healthy life. The problem with this research is that it classifies moderate drinking for women as consuming a standard drink most days. Our Australian society seems to promote binge drinking over moderate drinking, and this is linked with increased risks to health such as dementia, depression, liver disease, kidney disease, heart disease, digestive disorders and cancer. Remember this isn't a 30-day challenge, it's a lifestyle. I'm not asking you to quit drinking alcohol forever, I'm asking you to drink mindfully, if at all.

Sugar from soft drinks can be a trigger for hot flushes as well as promoting blood sugar imbalances. Soft drink with artificial sweeteners are not any better. It's time to stop the sugary soft drinks. If you miss bubbles, swap to sparkling water instead which you can flavour with many different things including lemons, limes, berries, pear, apple, cucumber or mint.

Good news! I'm not going to ask you to quit your morning coffee. There are health benefits of drinking coffee in moderation. That is, if your coffee is black and no sugar. Yes, its ok to add a little coconut oil or butter.

Additional benefits of coffee include:
- Is an antioxidant
- Increases alertness
- Increases cognitive function
- Can increase energy levels
- Improves mood
- Can help burn body fat
- May lower risk of Type 2 diabetes (if it doesn't contain sugar).

But don't overdo it!

My biggest concern with coffee is mould and mycotoxin contamination. Roasting coffee kills the mould but not the mycotoxin. Byron Bay Coffee Organic Espresso Blend, had undetectable mycotoxin levels at testing. Other brands that I'm aware of that have tested and passed include Bulletproof Coffee and Purity Coffee.

MENOPAUSE SUPERFOOD: PHYTOESTROGENS

Phytoestrogens are compounds found in plants that have an estrogen like effect in the body. They have a similar shape to oestradiol and have the ability to bind to and activate estrogen receptors. They are found in nuts (almonds, cashews, pistachios, walnuts), seeds (flaxseed/linseed, sesame, sunflower), legumes (chickpeas, black beans, mung beans, lentils, red kidney beans, spilt beans) garlic, rice, coffee, sprouts (alfalfa), fruit (apples, pomegranates, grapes, berries) and vegetables (broccoli, cabbage, celery, carrots, sweet potato).

Phytoestrogens can be further classified into isoflavones, stilbene, coumestan, and lignan.

Isoflavones are the most widely studied phytoestrogen and are mostly found in soy and legumes. There is a lot of talk about soy products. I personally do not recommend soy as most of it is genetically altered and highly processed these days. Soy is also goitrogenic. Goitrogenic foods can reduce thyroid function. Reduced thyroid function is linked with worsening menopausal symptoms. Resveratrol is found in grapes and peanuts and is the most common stilbene containing phytoestrogen. Coumestan containing foods include nuts, broccoli, cabbage and spinach. Flaxseed/linseed is the highest source of lignans. Peanuts, fruits, berries, vegetables, tea and coffee are other sources. Dietary phytoestrogens need to be metabolised by your digestive bacteria. Hence why it's so important to have a healthy microbiome. Your microbiome is your collection of good bacteria or probiotics. Without them you cannot break down your food or utilise your phytoestrogens. As phytoestrogens can bind to estrogen receptors, they are useful in cases of estrogen dominances (as can be found in perimenopause) as they are weaker than estrogen and can dilute the amount of free receptors available to bind to estrogen molecules. They are also useful in cases of low estrogen levels (post menopause) as they can bind to receptors and help increase the function of the available estrogen. Phytoestrogens can also reduce the risk of estrogen related cancers as they inhibit the action of cytochrome P450. This enzyme converts androgens to estrogens. Elevated cytochrome P450 is associated with breast, adrenal and endometrial cancers. It's a win-win scenario for all women.

Other benefits of phytoestrogens include:
- Improve general health and longevity via its action of being an antioxidant
- Reduces total and LDL cholesterol
- Reduces elevated blood pressure
- Reduces blood sugar and insulin levels
- Assists in weight loss by reducing visceral fat, improving leptin levels and suppressing appetite
- May improve bone density
- Helps maintain and improve cognitive function
- Reduces ageing of the skin

- Improves immune response and can reduce symptoms of allergy.

For more information about adding phytoestrogens to your diet, see the 7 day meal planner in the interactive version of the book.

Should I avoid anything? If you have any individual intolerances, it's important to cut these out of your diet permanently. The majority of women experience significant improvements when they remove grains and dairy. If you have never tried a grain and/or dairy-free diet, I highly recommend it.

GLUTEN IN GRAINS

There is no nutritious quality found in gluten containing food that can't be found in other foods. So, going gluten-free has no downside. Some women will say the downside is the lack of taste, and a decade ago I would have agreed, but today there are so many yummy gluten-free foods available. On the bright side, a growing number of people are noticing they feel significantly better without it. Symptoms that may be linked with gluten include any digestive discomfort—especially bloating, wind, skin itch, rash, brain fog and memory issues. Many people have immune reactions to gluten and this may be linked with autoimmune conditions. Did you know Alzheimer's is linked with undiagnosed Coeliac disease (gluten allergy)?

CASEIN/LACTOSE IN DAIRY

It is estimated 75% of the population cannot tolerate dairy. It's not surprising when you consider it's the perfect food for calves, but not humans. Humans are designed to consume human breast milk in infancy and even as a child our production of lactase (the enzyme that breaks down milk) is already starting to reduce. This is the reason why some women say they could tolerate milk as a child, but now it gives them an upset tummy.

Other signs of lactose intolerance include sinus congestion, headaches, joint pain, brain fog, skin itch and fatigue.

THE ULTIMATE CHECKLIST FOR INVINCIBLE EATING

1. It's important to allow your digestive system time to rest and digest. Ideally, there would be a minimum of 12 hours without food every day. This can be easily obtained if you finish dinner before 7 pm and do not have breakfast before 7 am. These hours can be moved around depending on your life, as long as there is a minimum 12 hours free from food.

2. Stop grazing. You should focus on eating meals and not constantly snacking. If you are hungry, consider having a drink.

3. Are you getting adequate fluid? Filtered water and herbal teas count towards your minimum 2 litres daily. Coffee in moderation is allowed, but as a diuretic, it doesn't count towards your water count.

4. Add in menopause-specific teas like sage, fennel and green tea to your daily routine.

5. Did you eat fruit today? Check your fruit intake, as it's an important source of fibre.

6. When planning your meal, start with the protein source. Good examples include fish, chicken, beef, lamb and eggs.

7. Do you want to add a salad or vegetables to your meal? Look at what's seasonally available. Is your garden abundant with leafy salad greens or is it time to pull out the winter vegetables?

8. Is there a good fat in the meal or do you need to add one? Some meals naturally contain a good fat source such a seafood dish, while others require more thought. You may want to drizzle some olive oil over the meal or add avocado to your dish.

9. Add in a daily serve of phytoestrogenic foods. LSA is a delicious and handy addition to most meals. LSA is ground

linseed (flaxseed), sunflower seeds and almond. You can sprinkle this over your salad. My daughter uses this as a coating on her homemade chicken schnitzel instead of breadcrumbs (see interactive guide for the recipe).

10. Leave space for soul food. This isn't a 30-day meal plan; it's a lifestyle. Life contains special events that deserve celebrating and moments where indulgence is wanted. Allow yourself two servings of guilt-free soul food a week.

11. If you can honestly say you are eating as described in this book, yet you have excess weight to lose or your weight loss has plateaued, the first step is to go back to point one above and reduce your feeding window. Dr Jason Fung's book, *The Obesity Code*, outlines the benefits of time-restricted feeding which includes weight loss and improving insulin sensitivity. The next goal would be 18-hour fasting window and 6-hour feeding window. I find it easiest to skip breakfast and start at lunch; many others have found it easier to skip dinner. It doesn't matter which meal you skip, what matters is the length of fasting window.

If you are reducing your feeding window, you might find these tips on reducing your appetite helpful:

- Avoid all artificial sweeteners as they can trigger hunger and insulin response
- Physically remove yourself from food and food smells
- Drink more water
- Stay busy
- Understand that hunger comes in waves and you only need to wait out the wave
- Drinking green tea or coffee can help.

Would you like a seven-day meal planner with recipes?
Head over to the interactive version for more.

v = vitamins and minerals

It's important to acknowledge that nutrient deficiencies do cause disease. For example, an iron deficiency causes anaemia and a vitamin C deficiency causes scurvy. Other drugs can be used as a band-aid so you won't feel as bad, but nothing (other than topping up the missing nutrient) can help restore health.

To be classified as a vitamin or mineral, the substance must be essential for health and your body must obtain this nutrient through the diet, as our body cannot produce it. Vitamins are organic and can be broken down by air, heat or water. Minerals are inorganic and hold on to their chemical form when exposed to the elements.

Some nutrients are water-soluble and other fat-soluble.
- **Water-soluble nutrients** are short-lived in the body and must be consumed daily to keep up adequate amounts. They are generally safe to take on an empty stomach as

they break down and absorb quickly with the water you swallowed them with.

- **Fat-soluble nutrients** can be stored in the body and have a long lifespan. These are generally better to take with food as they require a fat source present to be absorbed. Most fat-soluble supplements come with a small amount of oil to enhance usability.

Fat-soluble nutrients are more likely linked with complications from overconsumption, as the body can store them. Consider an overload of iron as an example. Iron is an essential mineral but having too much is as dangerous as having too little. Hence, I am a big fan of testing to make sure you find a happy medium for optimal health. In the section below I have noted possible concerns with overdosing.

Drug interactions can occur with supplementation. In some cases, they increase the need for the nutrients, in other cases they can reduce the need and may cause additional problems. I don't recommend self-prescribing. This information is provided as a guide and to assist as a conversation starter with your health care provider.

VITAMIN A
FAT-SOLUBLE
- Retinol
- Dihydroretinoid.

Beta carotene is NOT vitamin A. The carotenoid family is a provitamin. In the right conditions, it can be converted to vitamin A however these days, genetic testing has discovered that more and more people are missing specific enzymes necessary for this conversion and need to supplement with actual vitamin A. Genes to consider here include the BCM01 and BCM02 gene.

Food sources of vitamin A:
- Animal meat: liver, cod liver oil, egg
- Dairy products: ghee, butter, cheese.

Food sources of beta carotene:
- Fruit: rockmelon, apricot, papaya, mango
- Vegetables: sweet potato, carrot, broccoli, kale, dandelion, spinach, pumpkin, capsicum, tomato, peas.

Deficiency:
Deficiencies can be caused by low-dietary intake, vegetarianism, inability to convert beta carotene to vitamin A, inadequate fats in the diet or fat malabsorption (as it is a fat-soluble nutrient and needs fat to be absorbed), chronic exposure to toxins (such as cigarette smoke and alcohol) or zinc deficiency (as zinc is required for metabolism of vitamin A). Obese women are found to have lower levels of fat-soluble vitamins such as vitamin A.

Uses:
- Essential for vision, especially night vision and also needed for eye lubrication. Severe deficiency can lead to blindness.
- It has an important role to play with immune health and preventing autoimmune conditions, especially thyroiditis.

- It is important for healthy looking skin. Vitamin A deficiency has a role to play in acne and keratoinosis pilosis (white lumps on hair follicles on the back of the arms).
- Supports healthy teeth. Enamel issues can be due to lack of vitamin A.
- Needed for gene transcription.
- Essential for healthy mucous membranes (think vagina, digestion, sinus).
- Helps keep the brain young and flexible.
- Needed for cellular proliferation and tissue remodelling.
- Associated with improved hormonal status (estrogen and testosterone).
- Helps maintain bone mass.

Dangers:
Hypervitaminose A can be lethal, however highly unlikely unless you are an Arctic explorer eating the liver of polar bears.

Medication interactions:
- Vitamin A can increase the risk of bleeding when taken with blood thinners (e.g., warfarin).
- Avoid taking vitamin A with other retinoid drugs as they can increase your risk of toxicity.
- Medications that inhibit fat absorption such as Xenical, block the absorption of all fat-soluble nutrients including vitamin A.

Fun fact:
Exciting research is looking into the possibility of using vitamin A as a cancer treatment in the future.

VITAMIN B

B	Name	Key Words
1	Thiamine	• Major role in digestion. Helps produce hydrochloric acid so we can digest our food. Prevents constipation, regulates appetite • Brain health and the maintenance of memory • Nerve health.
2	Riboflavin	• Needed for energy production • Digestion of food and enhances the absorption of other nutrients • Essential for new cell production.
3	Niacin	• Digestion and detoxification • Nervous system and brain health • Beneficial for good moods and memory • Hair and skin health • Energy and sleep regulation • Cellular health and DNA repair.
5	Pantothenic	• Energy • Helps regulate stress and moods • Hormone production.
6	Pyridoxine	• Moods, especially anxiety • Is needed for over 100 different reactions in your body • Glucose regulation and energy production • Digestion, especially protein • Immunity and red blood cell formation.
7	Biotin	• Energy • Digestion: protein, carbs, and fats • Cell signalling and gene modification.
9	Folate*	• Essential for new cell production • Improves cardiovascular health • Reduces cancer risk • Improves cognitive function and mood.

12	Cobalamin	• Essential for healthy nerves • Essential for healthy blood and cardiovascular system • Energy producing • Mood and memory promoting • Digestion of protein carbohydrates and fats.

* Avoid folic acid forms of folate and foods fortified with folic acid. Throw out supplements with this form in it. Methyl folate or folinic acid are the preferred forms.

WATER-SOLUBLE

B vitamins play important roles within the body, both individually and collectively. It's best to always start with the entire B family, called a 'B complex'. and then add individual B vitamins if required later. B vitamins are water-soluble which means they dissolve in water. They are easily transported around the body but generally aren't stored—which means you need a daily intake of these nutrients.

The following healthy foods are good sources of B vitamins:
- Meat: red meat, poultry and fish
- Eggs
- Legumes and lentils
- Nuts and seeds
- Dark green leafy vegetables (broccoli, spinach)
- Fruits: citrus, banana, avocado.

Uses:
- Improving digestion
- Increasing energy
- Improving nerve health
- Essential for good heart health
- Better moods and memory
- Production of new healthy cells
- May help to prevent cancer.

Dangers:

Yellow urine. This is expected with vitamin B supplementation and stops when you stop supplementing. It is in no way dangerous; it's simply a by-product of B vitamin metabolism. Warning: it can be fluorescent!

Medication interactions:

- Proton pump inhibitors such as Nexium (esomeprazole) block B12. Supplementation is needed.
- Blood sugar regulating medication such as metformin reduce B12. Supplementation is needed.
- B vitamins especially B6 and B12 can help reduce symptoms associated with chemotherapy treatment with drugs such as capecitabine and fluouracil. Supplementation is beneficial but speak to your cancer specialist first.

Fun facts:

- B vitamin was once thought to be one vitamin, but further research discovered it was multiple nutrients. At one point, researchers thought it went all the way up to 20 nutrients.
- Choline was once called B4 until it was discovered that the body can produce small amounts of this nutrient —and lost its status as a vitamin. However, choline is not produced in large enough amounts by the body and is still essential to consume daily. It is still found in most B complexes. It's an essential nutrient for heart and brain health.
- Inositol was called B8 and was demoted for the same reason as choline. Inositol is important for digestion, blood sugar regulation and cravings. There is also research connecting inositol to better thyroid function.
- Other common nutrients once thought to belong here include: L-carnitine (B20) and dimethylglycine (B16).

VITAMIN C
WATER-SOLUBLE
- Ascorbic acid
- Mineral ascorbates (buffered vitamin C): sodium ascorbate, calcium ascorbate, potassium ascorbate, magnesium ascorbate, zinc ascorbate, molybdenum ascorbate, chromium ascorbate, manganese ascorbate
- Ascorbyl palmitate —better form for topical applications.

Companions:
Vitamin C is best utilised with additional bioflavonoids. Bioflavonoids are plant-derived antioxidants that give 'flavour' to plants. There are over 6000 known bioflavonoids. Some you may have heard of include quercetin, hesperetin, catechin, luteolin, cyanidin.

Food sources:
- Tropical fruit: guava, pawpaw, pineapple, kiwi
- Greens: spinach, brussel sprouts and broccoli
- Salads: capsicum, tomato and avocado
- All berries but strawberries are the highest
- Citrus fruit: oranges, lemons, grapefruit
- Durian: but you are not eating it at my house!

Deficiency:
People who don't eat enough fruit and vegetables are at risk of vitamin C deficiency. Heavy drinkers and smokers are also at an increased risk. Scurvy is caused by a severe vitamin C deficiency. It is characterised by bruising, bleeding gums, tiredness, skin complaints and can even result in death.

Uses:
- Vitamin C is needed for collagen formation. Good collagen levels are needed to maintain skin plumpness and reduce wrinkles. Vitamin C is also needed to keep muscles and bones healthy and keep teeth in your mouth.

- It helps reduce stress levels and anxiety while producing happy neurotransmitters and improving cognition.
- It is an antioxidant and can help protect the body from disease.
- Most known for its role in immunity. It helps prevent infections and helps overcome infections faster.
- Great for cardiovascular health and may lower blood pressure. It also assists with the absorption of iron and minimises anaemia.
- Reduces capillary fragility, which helps prevent bruises and easy bleeds.
- May help regulate hormones by decreasing FSH and increasing progesterone.

It's important to note menopausal women have an increased need for vitamin C.

Dangers:
Excess vitamin C is evacuated from the body in the form of diarrhoea. Ever eaten too much fruit?

Medication interactions:
Vitamin C may reduce the effectiveness of amphetamine medications such as adderall. It's best to talk to your prescribing doctor before taking vitamin C.

Fun fact:
Want to know how much vitamin C your body needs to reach saturation? There is a test called the vitamin C bowel tolerance test. Vitamin C is consumed and counted until diarrhoea begins. For example, you can take 1000 mg every hour and see how many hours you can go until you reach your tolerance. It's a good indication of how deficient you are in vitamin C. Benefits of doing this include increased energy, increased immunity, accelerated healing and improved detoxification. It's not recommended if you have high iron levels as it increases your iron absorption, or if you have digestive issues such as IBS (irritable bowel syndrome).

VITAMIN D

FAT-SOLUBLE NUTRIENT

- D2: ergocalciferol
- D3: cholecalciferol (most active form).

Companion:

Best to take with vitamin K.

Sources:

- Safe sunshine exposure (note, sunscreen blocks vitamin D absorption).
- Fatty fish, especially cod liver oil.
- Egg yolk.
- Mushrooms, especially those grown under ultraviolet light.

Deficiency:

Vitamin D deficiency is extremely common these days as people aren't getting adequate sun exposure or hiding under sunscreen and missing out on vitamin D. Women with fat malabsorption issues struggle to utilise this fat-soluble vitamin and women with a high body mass also struggle to get adequate vitamin D. Postmenopausal, your requirements for vitamin D increase.

Uses:

- Immune regulation—great for either an underactive or overactive immune system.
- Helps prevent cancer (especially colon, prostate, and breast).
- Strengthens bone.
- Reduces pain and inflammation. Several studies link decreased pain tolerance with lowered vitamin D levels.
- Plays a role in nerve health and may prevent or reduce MS (multiple sclerosis).
- It also plays a role in muscle health; deficiency can cause muscle cramps, spasms, and pain.
- Helps regulate the life of a cell (growth, repair, and death).

- May play a role in preventing Type 1 and Type 2 diabetes and regulating blood sugar levels.
- Plays a role in cholesterol and triglyceride management, blood pressure regulation and preventing cardiovascular disease.
- Keeps your brain, memory and cognition working well.

Medical Interactions:

- Using corticosteroid medication such as prednisone reduces your vitamin D levels. Supplementation is needed.
- Cholesterol reducing medication like cholestyramine or statins, reduce your vitamin D levels. Supplementation is needed.
- Fat absorbing medication such as Xenical (orlistat), reduces your vitamin D levels and supplementation away from this medication is required.
- Epilepsy medication such as phenytoin and phenobarbital, significantly reduce vitamin D levels. Supplementation is needed.

Fun fact:

There are vitamin D receptors in every cell and tissue of your body. From your brain to your toes—and all the bones, muscles and nerves along the way. Which means, it has a role to play in the health of your entire body!

VITAMIN E

FAT-SOLUBLE
- Tocopherol: alpha, beta, gamma, and delta
- Tocotrienol: alpha, beta, gamma, and delta.

Companion:
If you have any vitamin E supplements at home, please make sure they are balanced. Most supplements only contain alpha-tocopherol, which is only one source of the eight forms needed. Please only purchase oral products with all eight forms.

Sources:
- Seeds: sunflower
- Nuts: almonds, hazelnuts,
- Green vegetables: spinach, broccoli
- Fruit: kiwi, mango, tomato.

Deficiency:
Found in women on low-fat diets or those with digestion issues.

Uses:
- Specific nutrient for hormonal health.
- Specific nutrient for heart and general cardiovascular health.
- Helps prevent cancer.
- Helps to prevent/reduce all chronic disease.
- Enhances immune function.
- Good for eyesight issues as it's needed for a healthy retina and can reduce your risk of age-related macular degeneration and cataract formation.
- Plays a role in cognitive maintenance.
- Works as an antioxidant and protects against free radical damage.
- Topically to heal and lubricate mucus membranes (I often suggest vitamin E pessaries to women to reduce vaginal dryness and itch).

- Topically for haemorrhoids (vitamin E is also available as a suppository to help heal haemorrhoids).
- Topical for burns, chapped lips, reducing stretch marks and scars. Some people even say it helps reduce wrinkles.

Medication interactions:
- Do NOT take vitamin E with blood thinning drugs such as rivaroxaban, plavix, eliquis, aspirin or warfarin as they may increase your risk of bleeding. Check with your prescribing doctor if you are unsure.
- Do NOT take vitamin E if you are on HIV medication such as tipranavir, as it may increase your risk of bleeding.

Fun facts:
- Vitamin E was discovered in 1922 when researchers gave female rats a low vitamin E diet. All pregnant rats had litters that were stillborn. They later added lettuce and wheat germ (high vitamin E sources) and healthy babies were born.
- Vitamin E is so important for all stages of reproductive health. Menopause included.

VITAMIN K

FAT-SOLUBLE

- K1: phytonadione
- K2: menaquinones (MK4, MK7, MK9).

Companion:

Partners well with vitamin D.

Sources:

- Dark green leafy vegetables: spinach, broccoli, kale, lettuce
- Other vegetables: carrot, pumpkin
- Animal meat: poultry and swine
- Fermented foods: natto
- Nuts: pine nuts, cashews
- Egg.

Deficiency:

Generally, only found in women with fat malabsorption issues and some newborns as vitamin K is poorly transferred across the placenta and only found in low amounts in breast milk.

Uses:

- Is needed for blood clotting.
- Essential for bone, cartilage and muscle health.
- Improves dental health by carrying extra calcium and minerals into your teeth and strengthens bones.
- Prevents coronary heart disease by reducing calcification of the arteries. It also reduces the formation of varicose veins as increased calcification causes blood to pool in areas. It also plays a role in reducing stroke.
- Prevents and treats kidney disease by reducing calcification of the tubules and reducing the formation of kidney stones. Supplementing vitamin D without vitamin K increases your risk of kidney stones, so it's best to use these two in combination.

- May promote youthful skin by activating the Matrix-GLA and preventing calcification of elastin, which is needed to prevent saggy and wrinkles.
- It is being researched for its role in increasing insulin sensitivity and decreasing Type 2 diabetes.

Medication interactions:

- Vitamin K antagonist medications work to reduce blood clotting by reducing the action of vitamin K. Do not supplement with these medications. Warfarin is an example of a Vitamin K antagonist.
- Cholesterol lowering medication such as colestipol reduce all fat-soluble nutrients including vitamin K and supplementation should be taken away from this medication.
- Fat absorbing medications like Xenical, reduce all fat-soluble nutrients and supplementation is needed.

Fun fact:

There are 13 forms of K2 (MK1, MK2, MK3, etc.) but only three have been researched. I think this is exciting as there are still so many potential natural therapeutic substances out there that could restore health. This is where we should be spending our research dollars, not on drugs.

CALCIUM

FAT-SOLUBLE

- Calcium citrate
- Calcium orotate
- Calcium carbonate
- Calcium malate
- Calcium phosphate
- Calcium gluconate
- Calcium lactate
- Calcium oxide – avoid
- Hydroxyapatite.

Companion:

- Magnesium
- Vitamin D
- Vitamin K.

Sources:

- Vegetables: cabbage, kale, and broccoli
- Seeds: sesame, poppy, chia
- Nuts: almonds
- Sardines and salmon with bones
- Beans and lentils
- Dairy, although it's not a good source. Calcium from broccoli is about 100 times more absorbable than dairy and isn't linked with health complications such as cancer, that dairy is linked with.

Deficiency:

It can be a problem if you are on a low-fat diet. Diets high in oxalates can also be problematic as oxalates bind to calcium and make it less available.

Uses:

- Most famous for its role is bone health
- Dental health

- Needed for muscular contraction
- Vascular contraction and vasodilation (heart health). It may also reduce high blood pressure
- Nerve signalling
- Hormonal signalling
- Reduces risk of colon cancer.

Most women are not aware that there are dangers of over-supplementing with calcium.

These dangers are linked with supplementation and not with the consumption of calcium-rich foods—except dairy. Due to this, I often recommended dietary changes to improve calcium levels, or, if I do supplement, I include a companion nutrient such as magnesium to minimise these risks.

Dangers:
- Kidney stones and renal damage. Calcium oxalate is what most kidney stones are made of. If you tend to produce stones, avoid calcium supplementation altogether.
- A common cause of hyperparathyroidism.
- Constipation.
- Can reduce the absorption of other minerals, such as zinc and iron.
- Some studies are linking excess calcium supplementation to cardiovascular disease. Plaque caused by calcium deposits in the arteries (calcification) contribute to arterial stiffness and can interfere with valve function.

Medication interactions:
- Antacids like Nexium and Mylanta increase calcium loss via your urine. It's better to reduce your need for these drugs and increase calcium containing foods than to start supplementing.
- Laxatives can reduce calcium absorption. If you are on long term laxatives, it is a priority to fix your digestion, rather than add a calcium supplement.

- Glucocorticoids, like prednisone, are linked with osteoporosis caused by calcium depletion. Calcium should be co-prescribed when steroids are used for longer than a month.
- It's important to co-prescribe calcium with bisphosphonates medication for osteoporosis, although they can't be taken at the same time. Ideally, separate them by at least four hours.
- Do not take calcium with antibiotics such as fluoroquinolone as it reduces the effectiveness.
- Calcium may reduce levothyroxine's effectiveness if taken together. Ensure these are taken at different times of the day.
- Seizure medication like phenytoin, needs to be taken at least four hours before or after, calcium supplementation.
- Medication for Paget's disease such as tiludronate disodium need to be taken at a different time from calcium supplementation.
- Thiazide type diuretics increase calcium reabsorption; therefore, supplementation is NOT recommended.

Fun fact:
Calcium is the most abundant mineral in the body!

CHROMIUM

- Chromium chelate
- Chromium picolinate
- Chromium chloride.

Companions:
Vitamin B and C increase absorption of chromium.

Sources:
- Brewer's yeast
- Vegetables: broccoli, green beans
- Herbs and spices: garlic, basil
- Beef and poultry
- Fruit: apple, banana, grapes.

Deficiency:
Deficiency is very common.

Uses:
- Enhances the action of insulin, helps to regulate blood sugar levels and prevent diabetes.
- Can reduce cravings.
- Assists in carbohydrate, protein and fat metabolism.

  Small doses regularly are best to balance blood sugars.

Medication interactions:
Can potentiate metformin and make it more effective. Great addition if you are looking for an alternative to a dose increase, or if you are wanting to reduce your dose and still get a benefit.

Fun fact:
Chromium 6 (hexavalent) is the toxic form of chromium resulting from industrial pollution. It is the toxin that Erin Brockovich fought so hard to protect her community against.

COPPER

- Copper gluconate
- Copper amino acid chelates
- Cupric oxide
- Cupric sulfate

Sources:
- Shellfish: oysters
- Nuts: cashews, almonds
- Dark green leafy vegetables
- Black pepper
- Cocoa
- Yeast
- Copper cooking equipment.

Deficiency:
Toxicity is more common than deficiency. Rarely do my prescriptions include copper. I would need blood testing to confirm deficiency before I would recommend anyone take copper.

Uses:
- Copper is a building block for ceruloplasmin. Ceruloplasmin is needed for proper iron absorption. If you are having trouble absorbing iron, ask your doctor to check your copper and ceruloplasmin levels.
- Energy production: builds red blood cells
- Immunity: builds white blood cells needed to ward off invaders
- Copper conducts your nerves signals, much like how we use copper in industry
- Copper plays an important role in maintaining collagen and elastin—supporting major structural components of our bodies, preventing sagging skin and keeping bones strong and joints healthy.
- Copper is needed for healthy skin. Deficiency has been linked with depigmentation of the skin.

Dangers:

- Copper and zinc work in ratio with each other; too much of one knocks the other around. Elevated copper and low zinc are linked with estrogen dominance. Estrogen dominance enhances the growth of reproductive tissues, e.g., fibroids, polyps, endometriosis.
- Too much zinc and not enough copper may be linked to elevated cholesterol and cardiovascular disease.
- Elevated copper is linked with depression, social withdrawal, anxiety and memory issues.
- Copper imbalances are also possible causes of central nervous system issues like Multiple Sclerosis.
- May be linked with the development of diabetes.

Medication interactions:

There are currently 32 known drug interactions with copper. As copper is rarely prescribed, I haven't added the individual drugs here. If you are taking copper or thinking about starting, check that your prescribing health care professional has looked up its potential interactions.

Fun Fact:

Some people wear copper bracelets to help them with their arthritic pain.

IODINE
- Potassium iodide
- Sodium iodide.

Companions:
- Selenium
- Magnesium
- B2 and B3
- Vitamin C.

Sources:
- Seaweed: kelp, nori, kombu, wakame
- Seafood
- Eggs
- Salt: iodised salt is not recommended. Natural salt contains 43 trace minerals and is a super food. Iodised salt is highly processed and has had 40 of the minerals removed, imbalancing its nutrient profile.

Deficiency:
Goiter (swollen thyroid/neck) is one of the clinical signs of low iodine. It can also cause dysfunction in the production of thyroid hormones and can be linked to thyroid cancer.

Uses:
- It is an essential building block for thyroid hormone and needed for thyroid health. Your thyroid is responsible for controlling your metabolism.
- Essential for breast health and can be used to reduce breast pain, reduce fibrocystic breast disease and may even be protective against breast cancer.
- Mental acuity.

Dangers:

Don't take iodine if your thyroid dysfunction is immune based (e.g., Hashimoto's or Graves), unless under supervision of a health care professional as it can increase thyroid antibodies.

Medication interactions:

- Do NOT take iodine with hyperthyroid medication such as tapazole.

- Do NOT take iodine with ACE inhibitors or potassium-sparing diuretics as you must avoid potassium with these drugs and iodine potassium is the main form of iodine supplementation.

- Do NOT take iodine if you are on lithium, as it increases your risk of an underactive thyroid.

Fun fact:

Goitrogen containing foods can interfere with the uptake of iodine and exacerbate iodine deficiency. Foods high in goitrogens include soy, cabbage, broccoli, cauliflower and other cruciferous vegetables. Cooking these vegetables destroys their goitrogenic qualities.

IRON

Anaemia or low iron is common in menstruating women, whereas iron overload is common in postmenopausal women. Please test iron levels before starting an iron supplement and retest again later.

Forms:
- Heme: mostly meat
- Non-heme: mostly vegetarian sources.

Companions:
Vitamin C (add if low, avoid if high).

Sources:
- Meat: beef, lamb
- Seafood: oysters, clams, sardines
- Poultry: chicken, turkey
- Nuts: pistachios, cashews, almonds, brazil nuts, hazelnuts
- Beans: white beans, lentils, kidney beans, chickpeas
- Vegetables: spinach, broccoli, mushrooms.

Deficiency:
Symptoms of iron deficiency anaemia include fatigue, muscle cramps, restless legs, dizziness, rapid heartbeat, palpitations, headache, shortness of breath, insomnia, pale colour and concentration issues.

Toxicity:
Symptoms of iron overload include fatigue, joint pain, abdominal pain, irregular heartbeat, potential blood sugar issues, potential liver issues, depression and concentration/cognition issues.

Uses:
- Is a key building block of haemoglobin. Its job is to transport oxygen from the lungs to the tissues.
- Oxygenated tissues promote energy production.

- Is responsible for the normal cellular functions such as growth, development and repair.

Iron related disease:
- Hemochromatosis is a genetic condition where individuals store excessive amounts of iron. Think of iron overload as rust inside your body; it's a severe condition.
- Thalassemia is another genetic disorder involving iron. These individuals don't make enough haemoglobin and many need transfusions to survive.
- Medication interactions:
- Iron reduces the absorption of tetracyclines antibiotics. Do NOT take together.
- Iron reduces the absorption of levodopa, methyldopa and carbidopa. Do NOT take together.
- Iron may interfere with levothyroxine absorption. If needed, take at a different time of the day.
- Proton pump inhibitors can cause low iron levels by stopping absorption. You can take both but better at different times of the day.

Fun Fact:
Donating blood is the easiest way to reduce ferritin (stored iron) levels. Not only does it save your life, it saves the lives of three others too. Talk about a win-win situation.

MAGNESIUM

Forms:

- Magnesium citrate
- Magnesium glycinate
- Magnesium chelate
- Magnesium threonate
- Magnesium malate
- Magnesium chloride
- Magnesium sulfate
- Magnesium taurate
- Magnesium orotate
- Magnesium oxide: only use for severe constipation.

Companions:

- Potassium
- Calcium
- Vitamin D
- Vitamin K.

Sources:

- Dark green leafy vegetables: spinach, broccoli
- Legumes: black beans, kidney beans
- Nuts and seeds: almonds, cashews
- Fruit: avocado, banana
- Meat: chicken and beef.

Deficiency:

Common signs of low magnesium include eye twitches, leg cramps, headaches/migraine, anxiety/depression, poor stress tolerance and constipation.

Uses:

- Magnesium is an essential mineral cofactor in more than 300 enzymatic reactions.
- It is needed for muscular relaxation.

- The most important muscle in your body is your heart. This is an extremely important nutrient for heart health. It is needed for normal blood pressure and heart rhythm. It can reduce palpitations and angina.
- Very important for nerve impulse conduction.
- Helps regulate blood sugar levels; diabetics have a higher demand for magnesium.
- Magnesium is required for energy production.
- It contributes to the structural development of bone. Emerging evidence is looking at magnesium being more important than calcium regarding bone health.
- Is needed for new cell production due to its role in DNA and RNA replication.
- Is an important cofactor in the utilisation of glutathione. Glutathione is the master antioxidant.
- Essential for healthy happy moods, can help reduce the stress response and improve low moods such as anxiety and depression.
- May be useful in reducing all forms of pain.

Dangers:
Excess magnesium is not stored in the body. Therefore, excessive supplementation leads to short-term diarrhoea.

Medication interactions
- Magnesium may interact with bisphosphonates such as Fosamax, so it's best to take at different times of the day.
- Magnesium needs to be taken at least an hour away from antibiotics.
- Diuretics increase magnesium loss and increase the need for supplementation.
- Proton pump inhibitor like Nexium can cause magnesium deficiency by reducing absorption. Supplementation may be helpful.

- Magnesium may increase the effectiveness of diabetic medication and may allow for a lowering of dose. Insulin specifically reduces magnesium levels, so it's ideal to take a supplement with this drug.
- Magnesium supplementation may be needed with heart medications such as digoxin as it increases its excretion.
- Magnesium may interfere with levothyroxine, so it's best to take it at a different time of the day.
- Penicillamine can reduce magnesium. Taking additional magnesium at different times of the day can help reduce side effects of this drug.
- Corticosteriods such as prednisone increase your need for magnesium.

Fun fact:
This is my most prescribed nutrient and is also the easiest nutrient to increase, as it comes in so many options: pills, powders, creams, sprays and Epsom salt baths.

MANGANESE
Forms:

- Manganese gluconate
- Manganese sulfate
- Manganese ascorbate,
- Manganese amino acid chelate.

Sources:

- Brown rice
- Nuts: pecans, almonds
- Legumes: pinto, beans, navy beans, peanuts
- Fruit: pineapples, grapes, berries, kiwi.

Deficiency:

- Iron and manganese fight for absorption. If you have high iron stores, you will probably have low manganese levels.
- Carpel tunnel syndrome may be a sign of manganese deficiency.

Uses:

- Antioxidant—key component of manganese superoxide dismutase (MnSOD) the principle antioxidant inside your mitochondria.
- Helps with energy production as it optimises mitochondrial function (battery of your cell).
- Facilitates cartilage, tendon and bone development. Useful for osteoporosis and arthritis.
- Assists digestion of carbohydrates and in balancing blood sugar levels.
- Assists in protein digestion.
- Regulation of cholesterol.
- Is involved in the production of GABA (GABA promotes calmness, reduces anxiety, stabilises blood pressure and promotes restful sleep).
- Manganese is also called the 'brain mineral'. It may promote better memory.

- Plays a role in collagen formation and wound healing.
- Plays a role in sex hormone development.

Dangers:
- High manganese can cause iron deficiency anaemia.
- Inhaled manganese from industry goes straight to your brain and may cause permanent damage.

Medication interactions:
- Taking manganese alongside antibiotics may reduce the effectiveness of the antibiotics.
- Magnesium containing antacids and laxatives may reduce manganese levels.
- Iron supplementation may reduce manganese levels.

Fun fact:
Manganese is derived from the Greek word for magic.

MOLYBDENUM
Forms:
- Molybdenum trioxide
- Sodium molybdate
- Molybdenum chelate
- Ammonium molybdate.

Sources:
- Legumes: lentils, peas, beans
- Nuts: almonds, cashews, chestnuts
- Green leafy vegetables
- Eggs.

Deficiency:
Potentially linked with cancer.

Uses:
- Reduces elevated copper levels for people with Wilson's disease, as molybdenum and copper are antagonistic.
- Is needed to break down sulphur containing foods.
- Is an essential cofactor in the enzyme xanthine oxidase, which breaks down nucleotides and adds to the antioxidant capacity of the blood.
- Plays a role in detoxifying drugs and toxins.
- There are many things linked to Blue Zones[9] and molybdenum is just one. These are areas where the inhabitants tend to live longer than the general population, studies link higher levels of molybdenum in the soil and therefore the food, as being one possible reason for the extended life span.

Dangers:
- Not to be taken if you have a copper deficiency
- Toxicity may cause gout like symptoms.

---

9. https://www.bluezones.com

Medication interactions:

None known.

Fun fact:

Molybdemun is being used in pilot studies with promising results in cancer treatment for kidney, colorectal and breast cancer.

POTASSIUM

Forms:

- Potassium citrate
- Potassium chloride
- Potassium phosphate
- Potassium sulphate.

Companions:

- Sodium
- Magnesium.

Sources:

- Most fruit and vegetables: banana, potato, watermelon, tomato, sweet potato
- Legumes: lentils, kidney beans
- Meats: chicken, salmon, beef, turkey.

Deficiency:

Women who urinate often lose lots of potassium and this can start a vicious cycle of more urinating and more potassium loss.

Uses:

- Essential electrolyte.
- Potassium helps to regulate heartbeat.
- Needed for muscular health and nerve cell functions.
- Helps maintain a healthy blood pH level.
- Is needed for good kidney function and can help prevent kidney stones. Potassium is present in all body tissues and is required for normal cell function.
- Maintains intracellular fluid volume and transmembrane electrochemical gradients.
- Linked with healthy bones and muscles.
- Needs for blood glucose balance and stability in diabetes.

Dangers:

A severe potassium deficiency can be fatal.

Medication interactions:

- ACE inhibitors and angiotensin receptor blockers may cause potassium retention, so it's best not to take potassium with these drugs.
- Do NOT take potassium alongside potassium sparing diuretics.
- Loop and thiazide diuretics increase potassium excretion, so a potassium supplementation may be beneficial.

Fun fact:

Potassium is K on the periodic table. If you ever wondered why it's K and not P, I have the answer for you. K is short for kalium— the Latin name for potassium.

SELENIUM
Forms:
- Inorganic (selenate and selenite)
- Organic (selenomethionine and selenocysteine).

Companions:
- Vitamin E
- Vitamin B6.

Sources:
- Brazil nuts, cashews
- Seafood, meats, poultry
- Garlic
- Asparagus
- Eggs.

Deficiency:
The selenium content of food depends on whether the crop was grown in selenium-rich or poor soil and whether the animal meats were fed rich or poor selenium containing food. Unfortunately, Australian soils are naturally low in this mineral.

Uses:
- Essential for healthy thyroid hormone metabolism.
- Needed for glutathione peroxidase production—the master antioxidant, the cellular protector against oxidative damage.
- Major role in detoxification, especially helpful in removing mercury, arsenic, lead and cadmium.
- Helps regulate the immune system, prevents cancer and helps improve outcomes for people living with HIV.
- Selenium protects against chromosomal damage, stimulates DNA repair.
- Important nutrient for cardiovascular health.
- Deficiency may play a role in the development of cataracts and premature ageing in general.

- Selenium is needed to maintain good levels of cognition into later life.

Dangers:
Excess selenium can be problematic from excess hair loss to gastrointestinal upsets, breathing difficulties and cardiac problems.

Medication interactions:
Chemotherapy drug cisplatin increases selenium excretion. Selenium supplementation alongside cisplatin can help reduce side effects caused by this medication, so it's best to speak to your oncology specialist to determine dose.

Fun fact:
Selenium was discovered in 1817 and was named after the ancient Greek moon, Selene.

SILICA
Forms:
- Colloidal silica
- Silicon dioxide.

Companions:

Calcium and vitamin D for osteoporosis.

Sources:
- Banana
- Spinach and green beans
- Seafood
- Root vegetables
- Nuts.

Deficiency:

Deficiency is likely if you have had your stomach removed (gastrectomy).

Uses:
- To strengthen bones and prevent osteoporosis.
- For healthy hair, skin and nails.
- To reduce your risk of cardiovascular disease and stroke.
- To promote a strong memory.
- Good for treating sprains and strains.
- Can improve digestive function.

Dangers:

None know.

Medication interactions:

None known.

Fun fact:

Beer is a high source of silica; a schooner is almost three-quarters of your daily silica requirement! (Please don't view this as a recommendation to drink lots of beer, it's just a fun fact.)

SODIUM

WATER-SOLUBLE
Forms:
- Sodium chloride
- Sodium bicarbonate.

Companions—the other electrolytes:
- Potassium
- Magnesium
- Calcium.

Sources:
- Natural sea salt, e.g., Celtic sea salt is a superfood. It contains 43 trace minerals including sodium in the correct ratio. Table salt or iodised salt are not good options as they have been processed and the other nutrients have been removed, causing an imbalance.
- Seafood, seaweeds.

Deficiency:
Can occur if eating a low-salt diet or if you are an excessive sweater.

Uses:
- Maintains extracellular fluid volume.
- Facilitates nerve impulses.
- Regulates heartbeat and blood pressure. Deficiency can trigger dizziness and postural hypotension.
- Regulates muscle control and is a useful addition to prevent leg cramps.
- Regulates respiration and oxygenation.
- Plays a role in digestion. Deficiency can cause nausea.
- Improves immunity. It is antimicrobial, so great as a mouth gargle, sinus rinse and even topically for open sores (although may sting a little).

- Brain function. Low sodium has been shown to increase cognitive decline.

Dangers:

Too much sodium is also a problem—everything must be in balance. High levels are common in diets high in processed foods.

Medication interactions:

- Do NOT take sodium with lithium as it reduces its effectiveness.
- Do NOT take sodium with tolvaptan as it increases sodium levels.

Fun Fact:

Salt rooms are taking off around the world. By sitting in a room filled with salt, it opens up your lungs, improves skin health, energy and relaxation. Professional athletes go to salt rooms to enhance their abilities.

ZINC

Forms:

- Zinc sulphate
- Zinc gluconate
- Zinc acetate.

Companions:

Other antioxidants such as vitamin C.

Sources:

- Seafood, especially oysters
- Meat and poultry
- Nuts: cashews, almonds
- Legumes: chickpeas and kidney beans, although these contain phytates that may prevent zinc absorption

Deficiency:

Vegetarians are often deficient, as the highest zinc containing foods are animal products. Another issue is that vegetarian diets are high in copper, and copper and zinc compete against each other. Excessive alcohol consumption also reduces your zinc status.

Uses:

- Involved in over 100 processes in the body.
- Builds immunity.
- Improves hormonal balance and encourages progesterone production.
- Is a key building block for healthy skin and wound healing.
- Needed for protein synthesis.
- Needed for DNA replication and the development of new cells.
- Needed for the maintenance of healthy bones.
- Essential for the sense of taste and smell.
- May delay the progression of macular degeneration and age-related vision loss.

Dangers:

- Iron and zinc compete for absorption. If you are taking both vitamins, they need to be taken at different times of the day for optimum effects.
- Some women can't tolerate zinc on an empty stomach. When taken on an empty stomach it encourages higher absorption, however in some cases this causes nausea, headaches and an upset stomach. If you are sensitive to zinc, please take with a meal.

Medication interactions:

- Zinc may reduce your absorption of antibiotics, so it's best not to take at the same time.
- Ace inhibitors decrease zinc levels, so it's a good idea to supplement.
- Desferal medication removes excess iron from the blood, however it also removes zinc. Supplementation with zinc may be warranted.
- It is not advised to take zinc alongside immune suppressing medications such as prednisone.
- Penicillamine reduces your zinc levels, so it may be worth supplementing.
- Chemotherapy drug cisplatin reduces zinc levels, so it's best to speak to your oncologist about doses.
- Potassium sparing diuretics like amilloride increase zinc levels. Do NOT take together.
- Thiazide diuretics increase zinc excretion, so supplementing may be beneficial.

Fun fact:

Zinc is thought to have aphrodisiac qualities. It's due to the zinc in oysters that they are so popular with romantics.

Jennifer is sharing more in her
INTERACTIVE book.

See exclusive, behind-the-scenes
videos, audios and photos.

DOWNLOAD free content and go
From Invisible To Invincible.

deanpublishing.com/invincible

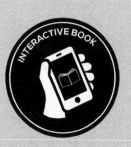

i = investigate

Women often have similar symptoms during this time, but very different underlying causes. Testing helps to determine why you are feeling the way you are and what individual treatment strategies you need to get back on track. Your doctor may be happy to run some of these tests for you under Medicare/NHS or your private insurance or you may have to pay for some of them privately. Not all of these tests are necessary for everyone. Some of these are functional tests and are not available from your doctor. Functional tests are available from integrated doctors and naturopaths.

BLOOD

- **Vitamin B12:** B12 deficiencies increase as we age and can cause numbness tingling in your hands and feet, balance difficulties, confusion, depression, fatigue, weakness, shortness of breath, heart palpitations, insomnia and anaemia.
- **Vitamin D:** This common deficiency causes fatigue, depression, muscle pain, poor immunity, pain and osteoporosis.
- **Copper:** High copper contributes to emotional withdrawing or isolating yourself, anxiety, poor stress response, stuttering,

memory issues, concentration issues, impaired learning, hyperactivity, depression, phobias, panic attacks, nervousness, schizophrenia and hyperactivity. Low copper may be the cause of anaemia or elevated cholesterol.

- **Zinc:** Low zinc can cause fatigue, poor immunity, skin problems, digestive issues, insomnia, poor taste and smell, allergies, poor appetite, hair loss, cognition issues and loss of libido. It's important to test copper and zinc together so you can determine their ratio. Ideal ratio is 0.7 units of copper to 1 unit of zinc.
- **Ferritin/iron:** This one could go either way. Some women in perimenopause have heavy periods and low iron stores and in post menopause when menstruation has ceased, high ferritin can become an issue. The most common sign is fatigue. Low ferritin can also cause weakness, irritability, leg pain, dizziness, headaches, ringing in your ears and shortness of breath.
- **Glucose/Insulin and HbA1c:** indicate problems with blood sugar regulation, abnormalities here are very common
- **CRP and ESR:** inflammatory markers that give us an indication of the amount of systemic inflammation in your body.
- **CA125:** is a specific marker for uterine inflammation and growths such as endometriosis, fibroids and polyps. It may be a useful marker to predict reproductive cancer risk.
- **Homocysteine:** this marker identifies cardiovascular disease risk and methylation issues.
- **Liver function test:** this test shows how well your liver is performing and if it is a fatty liver.
- **Thyroid testing:** TSH and thyroid antibodies are the most important, but try to have FT3, FT4, rT3 included as well.
- **Viral Panel Premium:** this test looks at various viral infections and can detect previous and current infections. Includes EBV, varicella, CMV, HSV1, HSV2 and HH6. These are all part of the herpes family and remain in your

system for life. Flare ups can cause similar symptoms to those experienced in menopause.

URINE

- **Urinary iodine status:** Low iodine levels cause breast pain and may increase your breast cancer risk. It is also related to an increased risk of osteoporosis and hypothyroidism. All conditions have an increased risk in post menopause.
- **GPL-TOX profile:** this test looks for 172 non-metal, toxic, environmental chemicals in your body, e.g., phthalates, benzenes, organophosphates.
- **Organic Acids test:** this test looks at intestinal dysbiosis, energy production, nutrient cofactor requirements and neurotransmitter metabolism. It pairs very well with genetic testing.

HAIR

HTMA: this test investigates for toxic metals in your body, such as mercury, lead, aluminium and cadmium. It also looks at mineral status and the ratios between the minerals and the metals.

SWABS

- **Genetic testing:** Have you had an ancestry test to look at your family tree? Were you aware this test gives you much more data than your family tree? You can also download your raw DNA code. It looks like lines and lines of random letters but put this through a translator site and you can unlock so many clues to your health and prevent potential complications down the track.
- **Microbiome testing:** This test investigates the health of your microbiome (collection of micro-organism). It is looking to

see if you have enough good bacteria and whether you have any problematic ones.

• MARCoNS (Multiple antibiotic resistant coagulase negative staphylococci): Essential if you have a history of mould exposure and are now experiencing fatigue and hormonal imbalance. There is further mould and biotoxins testing that can be performed if this is a potential area of concern.

You're probably very surprised that I haven't included any hormonal testing here.

What, no FSH, LH, estrogen, progesterone, testosterone or AMH? No, because it's normal for them to fluctuate on a daily basis and there is no current test that diagnoses menopause. The diagnosis comes 12 months after your last period. Your signs and symptoms indicate a problem, and we start by ruling out all other possibilities; treating them and then re-assessing whether we need to work directly with your hormones.

It surprises many women that they don't need hormonal support. Remember, some women breeze through menopause without a single symptom, and yet they still stop menstruating and their hormones drop. It's not always a hormonal issue, but the other factors that exasperate the changes at this point.

The earlier you can start working on your diet and lifestyle factors, the easier the transition will be. Maybe you will be one of those women that breeze straight through.

In the interactive book, I discuss additional tests, lab reference ranges and the ideal results for these tests.

n = non-toxic environment

'Multiple chemical sensitivity is diagnosed in 1% – 6% of the population, primarily affects middle age women, and is characterised by a broad range of symptoms involving multiple organ systems from headaches and fatigue to brain fog (confusion, depression, dizziness, memory problems), shortness of breath, nausea and muscular aches and pains.'
— *Nicole Bijlsma, Healthy Home Healthy Family*

Mmm...this sounds similar to menopausal symptoms. Even if you're not experiencing any of these, please do not skip this section. Toxins are everywhere and in everyone, don't think you are the exception. Even if you don't think they are affecting you now, they are slowing down your metabolism and liver function, altering your hormones and may produce symptoms in the near future.

This is not surprising when you consider there are over 140 million chemicals registered and most of these have never been tested to determine their safety for human exposure. It's a ticking time bomb for our world population.

The scary part is this:
Your home is probably your biggest source of toxicity!

Homes are filled with hormone-disrupting chemicals. Hormone disruptors are chemical substances that are found in the environment. Once in your body, they alter the way your hormones act.

Below are just a few easy lifestyle changes that can significantly reduce the amount of chemicals you are exposed to.

- **Organic sanitary products and incontinence pads.** If you are still menstruating, make sure you are using organic sanitary products. Have you ever considered how safe your female hygiene products are? The skin in and around your vagina is even more sensitive and permeable than skin in other areas. Here are a few examples of what you can find inside your average sanitary product: herbicides, pesticides, bleaches, plastics like BPA, phthalates, petrochemical additives, fragrances and even dyes (think coloured tampon string). The couple of extra dollars you spend on organic products are well worth the investment.

- **Phase out plastic containers and cling wrap.** These contain BPA or BPS (a BPA alternative which is just as bad). Replace your plastic containers with glass ones. Move leftover food into glass containers and you won't need cling wrap anymore. Don't forget to upgrade your water bottle at the same time. Glass or stainless steel are good options.

- **Avoid non-stick pots and pans.** Throw out your old non-stick pots and pans as these release toxic chemicals like

PFOS (perfluorooctanoic acid). If you have any aluminium cookware, put that in the bin too. Cast-iron pans, ceramic pots and stainless steel are the safest options.

- **Avoid flame retardants.** These are all over our homes. They are found in our lounges, mattresses, car seats, pillows, computer, television and even our pyjamas. These chemicals easily escape into our household dust. I know it's out of most people budgets to replace all these items, but by wet wiping instead of dusting and vacuuming with a powerful cleaner with HEPA filter, can dramatically reduce the number of contaminants in our homes. If you are in the market for new furniture, look for leather, cotton or wool products, as they generally contain no or low amounts of flame retardants.

- **Avoid fragrances.** Fragrances are hidden everywhere; they are not just in perfume. Think skin care, hair care or air fresheners. They may smell nice, but they could be any blend of over three thousand toxic chemicals. There is a loophole in labelling laws that allow companies to list fragrances because the scent is said to be their trademark secret. But as a consumer, you have no idea what is in the product or how toxic it may be. Fragrances can be absorbed via the skin, as is the case with skin care products, or absorbed via the nasal passage. Either way, this toxic combination of chemicals is wreaking havoc on your hormones.

- **Replace personal care products and cleaning products with chemical-free versions.** Shampoo, conditioner, body wash and other personal care products all contain nasty chemicals such as phthalates. Dr Mercola[10] calls phthalate 'gender benders' because of their direct effect on the reproductive system. Don't forget to change your toothpaste while you are at it. Toothpaste

---

10. https://www.mercola.com

can contain several nasties like parabens, SLS, triclosan and fluoride. Do this with your makeup as well—consider natural mineral-based products. Research a local low-toxic hairdresser to discuss safer hair dye options. Deodorant is worth a special mention as varieties that contain aluminium are toxic. The aluminium interferes with estrogen receptors, and this has been linked with breast cancer. Cleaning products are just as toxic, if not worse. Make sure you also avoid bleach containing products as they are well known hormone disruptors. When researching which new products to buy, look at the Environmental Working Group website (www.ewg.org). In the interactive version I have listed a few of my preferred brands.

- **Look at your sunscreen.** It comes in three main forms. Chemical filter, mineral filter and a combination of both. Five of the six most common chemical filters for sunscreen (4-MBC, OMC, OD-PABA, Bp-3, HMS) have been shown to exert significant estrogenic activity, which has been linked to breast cancer, hot flushes and fibroids. Mineral filters such as zinc oxide or titanium dioxide do not contain these nasty chemicals and have not been shown to have an estrogenic effect. Therefore, they are the safest option. Alternatively, my family and I don't use sunscreen at all. We have safe sun exposure and then cover up with hats, shirts and seek shade under a tree. Luckily, we have olive skin and this works well for us. Burning is not an option.

- **Stop using antibacterial products.** The main ingredient, Triclosan, has been banned overseas but not in Australia. It is a potent hormone disruptor.

- **Consider your clothing.** Invest in natural fibre clothing like cotton, bamboo, wool, silk or hemp and avoid synthetic fibres like polyester, nylon, rayon, acrylic, spandex and vinyl. Try to avoid clothes with crease reducing agents, flame retardants, stain repellent, are waterproof or need to be dry cleaned. When washing, use a low toxic detergent and don't use fabric softeners in your washing. Also, wash new clothes before wearing. For best results clothes need sunlight exposure.

- **Don't use weed killers.** The main ingredient, glyphosate, has been in the media a lot lately due to its toxicity. It damages our DNA, alters our hormone production and has been linked with estrogen dependant cancers such as breast cancer. Several countries have banned its use, but unfortunately, it's still available and highly used in Australia. Pull your weeds up the old fashion way with a little elbow grease and petition your local council to stop using these chemicals in our parks and playgrounds.

- **Eat as much organic food as you can afford.** Commercially grown foods contain herbicides, pesticides and other nasty surprises. Glyphosate, as mentioned above, is one of the most significant problems with eating commercially grown food, as it can't be washed off. It roots itself in the plant's DNA and there it stays. *What's with Wheat*, is a fabulous documentary which talks about this problem in great detail. Another option is to grow your own veggie patch or even better, convince someone else to get growing also and swap produce.

- **Filter your water.** It has been said the average glass of water has already passed through seven sets of kidneys and the number of residue medications (especially oral contraceptive pills) now in our water supply is scary. Buy a unit that filters at a minimum of 0.5 microns, my filter at home is an Aqua Pure[11] and it filters 0.2 microns. The lower the microns, the better.

11. 3M, 2019. https://www.3m.com.au

EXTRA TIPS FOR A HEALTHY HOME WITHOUT DISRUPTIVE SUBSTANCES

- **Get tough on dust.** Dust with a damp microfiber cloth, spring clean out any clutter, don't wear outdoor shoes inside the house, vacuum with a HEPA filter vacuum cleaner.
- **Minimise dust mites.** Dust mites are one of the most common allergens. They live in carpets, bedding, soft furniture, curtains, and stuffed toys. Consider swapping carpets for floorboards, curtains for blinds, sunning your mattress or updating it with a dust mite resistant version.
- **Ditch your microwave.** Radiation source and increases the bacterial content of food and reduces the nutrition value.
- **No smoking.** Don't allow anyone to smoke in or near your home or car.
- **Mould.** Consider testing your home for mould—especially if you live in a water-damaged house as not all mould can be seen or smelt. Most people related mould exposure to respiratory issues such as sinusitis, but did you know it can also cause fatigue, weakness, aches and pains, headaches, vision issues, digestive problems, cognitive decline, brain fog, sensitive skin, mood swings, issues with temperature regulation and flushing, excessive thirst, metallic taste, increased urination, electric shock, tingling and dizziness. Sounds very similar to menopause!
- **Go green inside.** Buy lots of indoor plants! Building biologist, Nicole Bijlsma, recommends 15 plants in a 140 m2 home. Her research found plants balance humidity levels, reduce chemical emissions, reduce airborne mould and bacteria, absorb carbon dioxide and release oxygen.

This section on living in a non-toxic environment wouldn't be complete without talking about the elephant in the room: radiation. Our daily exposure to radiation is increasing exponentially!

Just by sitting in the sun or placing our feet on the ground we are being exposed. While this exposure has evolved us in some ways to live, the amount and the intensity of new radiation sources around us is scary. We can't go back in time, but we should be avoiding and minimising certain sources.

Let's start by considering what radiation sources we are exposed to:

- Electrical devices in our home, e.g., mobile phones, smart devices, computers, cordless devices, entertainment units, fridge and microwave.
- Modern energy saving devices (such as fluorescent light bulbs), repeatedly interrupt the flow of energy. This pulsing of energy can create 'dirty electricity' or electromagnetic fields (EMF).
- In almost any location you can search for Wi-Fi and find multiple sources. Sitting in my home writing this, I have 12 different options to choose for Wi-Fi. OK, I don't have my neighbours' passwords, but I am being exposed to 11 extra sources of Wi-Fi that aren't mine and I can't switch them off. This is going to get worse with 5G on its way, as the strength of the radiation is increasing.
- Power lines and mobile phone towers.
- Radio waves from AM and FM radio.
- Medical imaging, e.g., x-rays.
- Flying.

Tips to reduce your exposure:

- Swap wireless devices for wired devices where possible. If you can't live without your home Wi-Fi, put it on an automatic timer so it switches off every night.
- Get some distance between you and your devices. Charge your device in an area away from you. Don't put phones in your pockets or bras. Use air tube headphones.

These headphones are specifically designed to reduce radiation. As my preferred brand changes as new ones come to market, see the interactive version for current recommendations.

- Turn your phone onto airplane mode overnight or leave it in another part of your home.
- Remove electrical devices from your bedroom, e.g., alarm clock, television, computer.
- Turn devices off at the wall when they are not in use.
- Don't put laptops on your lap!
- Don't have unnecessary x-rays.
- How necessary is your flight? Consider other forms of transportation or consider buying a few anti-radiation products.

Radiation reducing products:
- EMF filter to reduce dirty electricity
- Armor belly blanket (https://bellyarmor.com/collections/belly-blankets)
- Q-link products (https://www.shopqlink.com/)
- Mini radonex (https://www.rayonex.co.uk).

Supplements to reduce the effects of radiation:
- Vitamin C protects against iodising radiation damage.
- Ginkgo biloba contains flavonoids that protect against the formations of clastogenic factors (also known as chromosome breakage factors). These occur in the blood of people exposed to radiation. Foods that contain flavonoids include green tea, grape seed extract, blueberries, cherries, raspberries and blackberries.
- Other antioxidants that have been shown to reduce the damage caused by radiation include selenium, n acetyl cysteine, alpha lipoic acid, vitamin E and Co Q10.

Resources to consider:

- *Zapped*, by Ann Louise Gittleman, outlines 1268 ways to reduce your radiation exposure.[12]
- Documentary *Generation Zapped*.[13]

12. Gittleman, A.L. (2011). Zapped. HarperOne. https://annlouise.com/books/zapped
13. Zapped Productions, 2014-2017. https://generationzapped.com/resources

c = *contribution*

When comparing cultures that embrace menopause, as opposed to the Western culture that tries to avoid or delay menopause, one of the big differences is contribution.

When you step up into the wise woman role, you step up in the eyes of society. You have a more meaningful role in your community. Your life has a purpose, and your existence enhances the lives of others. But what is really interesting is that contributing also reduces your mortality rate. *The Berlin Aging Study*[14] found that looking after grandchildren reduces your mortality rate by 37%. This reduced mortality rate also included non-grandparents and childless older adults who looked after other people's grandchildren. It's a win-win situation.

Humans aren't the only species that benefit from looking after their grandkids. Whales and humans are the only species that don't die shortly after losing their fertility. We have a

14. The *Berlin Aging Study* is a multidisciplinary investigation of people aged 70 to over 100 years. The main study ran between 1990–1993 and included 516 individuals who were closely examined in 14 sessions. Sessions covered their mental and physical health, psychological functioning and social and economic situation. The study has continued as a longitudinal study, and surviving participants have been re-examined seven times since the initial study.

third of our lifespan still in front of us, and possibly more! One reason for this is that non-fertile women play a crucial role in society. Both in helping to raise grandkids and to help lead society in general. The oldest female whale is the one that leads the pod.

If you feel your life needs more purpose and you're interested in contributing, here are a few ideas to get you started.

VOLUNTEER YOUR TIME

- Reach out to a local animal shelter and see if they need help.
- Local schools are always after volunteers to help with reading programs, canteen, religion/ethic classes, etc.
- There are so many charity events you can participate in, such as the Sydney City to Surf fun run, as either a volunteer or a runner! Both roles are contributing.

SHARE YOUR KNOWLEDGE

- Do you have an interest in arts, tourism or history? Many museums, historical locations, and tourist areas need volunteers to help educate people about the area of interest.
- Mentor an up-and-coming person in your field.
- Start a support group.

RESPONSIBLE TRAVEL

This is a favourite of mine and something I regularly do. If you would like to join me on my next life-changing adventure, sign the expression of interest form in the interactive book.

- Once while holidaying in Vietnam, I volunteered in a local orphanage. Although I went to play with the older kids, due to my knowledge I ended up looking after the high-demand babies and children affected by Agent Orange.

- Gibbon Rehabilitation in Thailand[15] is on my list of places to return to. They prefer volunteers to stay three months due to the amount of training needed to look after the animals.
- I'm actively involved with Hands Across the Water—an Australian charity that financially supports orphanages around Thailand.[16] Twice I have been sponsored to ride my bike from Bangkok to Khao Lak. It's a five-day adventure. This experience was amazing; the comradery from the other riders and seeing the joy in the children at the orphanage at our final destination, was one of the best things I've ever done in my life.

Click the link in the interact book to see the video of this journey.

DONATE YOUR MONEY

- Consider sponsoring someone who is actively trying to make a difference.
- Donate directly to causes you are interested in.
- Buy from environmentally earth-friendly companies. Avoid buying products from companies that are destroying our planet to make a quick buck.

15. The Gibbon Rehabilitation Project, 1992 – 2019. https://www.gibbonproject.org
16. Hands Group, 2017. https://www.handsgroup.org.au

i = intuition

The dictionary describes intuition as *'the ability to understand something instinctively, without the need for conscious reasoning'* or *'a thing that one knows or considers likely from instinctive feeling rather than conscious reasoning.'*

We are all born with intuition. Some call it a gut feeling. It's interesting that it's called a gut feeling because your digestive system produces more neurotransmitters then your brain does. Your gut truly has a brain of its own, and it often guides us to make the right decisions. The menopausal transition is when this really comes alive. Now, more than ever is the time to sit and listen to what your body is telling you.

During menopause, we transition more into the right hemisphere of our brain. The creative side of our brain. It's now that we may rekindle our interest in arts and crafts, you may pick up your old knitting needles or find a nice spot to paint or take photos. But the right hemisphere is also about intuition, and with the transition into menopause, this creates a stronger more intense sense of knowing. Intuition can come from past experiences and accumulated knowledge from over your lifetime which may be conscious or unconscious. It's this strong connection to simply knowing something, without the need for evidence, that really provides wisdom if you choose to listen to it.

Health is a great example. No one knows YOUR body better than you! If you know something is wrong then don't accept anyone, doctors included, saying that it's simply the ageing process.

Listen to the body. It will provide you with countless answers and if you're not willing to listen now, it will only get louder and louder. In other words, your body may produce more pain or increase the number of issues you have until you take notice.

We have all had that friend or family member who knew something was wrong with them but didn't take action. Often, it's all too late and they regret it. Don't be that person. Symptoms are signs that something isn't right and often it's an easy fix—like a glass of water for a dehydration headache. But the longer you leave it, the more complicated it gets.

Listen to yourself more often and you will find out what's really important to you, rather than what society wants of you. You may feel pressure from society to be a certain way, but now is the time to make your own rules and go your own way. You have one opportunity to live this life, make it the one that lights you up and brings you joy.

If you would like to deepen your level of intuition, start by slowing down and becoming more mindful, remove all the stimulation, expand your practice of meditation and breathe work. Which leads straight into our next chapter...

b = breathe

Have you ever noticed that when you're relaxed you breathe slower? And when you're stressed you breathe faster, shorter breaths? Later in this chapter, I will walk you through two breathing exercises...but before that, let's talk about stress.

When you get stressed your body produces several stress hormones called cortisol, noradrenaline and adrenaline. These stress hormones can increase your core body temperature. This can trigger hot flushes as a way of getting rid of this excess heat. Have you noticed that stressful situations trigger hot flushes for you?

Other problems associated with elevated cortisol levels and menopause include:
- accelerated bone loss and links with osteoporosis
- blood sugar imbalances and increased risk of diabetes.

The adrenal glands are responsible for producing your stress hormones and are also responsible for creating the hormone precursors (androstenedione and DHEA). These precursors are needed for the conversion of your sex hormones (estrogen and testosterone), after your ovaries stop functioning. Therefore, it seems reasonable to assume optimal adrenal gland functioning is a necessity for a smooth menopausal transition.

Where possible, identify the stressors. Can they be removed, or do you need to manage them? In the case of unavoidable stress, like a sick family member, increase your stress management techniques. The best stress management tool is regular exercise and healthy eating. After this, consider talking to a trained professional—either a counsellor, psychologist or life coach. Emotional freedom technique, meditation, acupuncture and massage are also very helpful. Learning a few deep breathing techniques and practicing them regularly is one of the cheapest and most effective options.

Consider adding these supplements during times of continual stress:

- Vitamin C
- Vitamin B complex
- Magnesium
- Adaptogenic herbs. These herbs help you adapt to your situation and reduce your stress response. Here are a few examples: kava, rehmannia, licorice, ginseng, rhodiola, withania.

BREATHE EASY WITH BREATHWORK

The simple act of breathing allows us to oxygenate our body and calm our mind.

When you watch a newborn baby breathe, you will notice its tummy rise and fall; this is the way breathing should be. Over your lifetime, have you turned into a shallow breather or have you remained a deep breather?

A simple exercise is to sit in front of a mirror, place one hand over your stomach and the other over your chest.

When you take a big breath in, which hand moves first—the top or bottom hand? If you said the top hand, you are a shallow breather. If you said the bottom hand, you are still a deep diaphragmatic breather. We all start as diaphragmatic breathers, however life, poor posture and stress can sometimes train you into being a shallow breather.

Focus on the lower hand, really emphasise breathing into it. For many women, this is very foreign to them. This is where I want you to stay and focus until it becomes easy. Aim to try this every day for two to five minutes until you have retrained yourself to breathe this way, naturally.

If you have nailed this, move on to observing the timing of your breath. Do you naturally breathe in or out longer or are they the same? Count the seconds.

For optimal relaxation, the out breath should be longer.

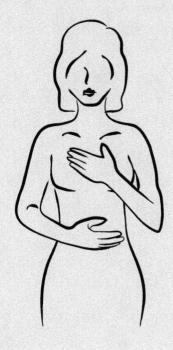

THE 7/11 BREATH

The 7/11 breath is a very helpful exercise. You simply count to seven on the in-breath and count to 11 on the out-breath. For some, this is too long, and it's OK to slowly work up to this number. As long as your exhalation is longer than your inhalation, you are on the right track.

This is the ideal exercise to do morning and night, to start and finish your day well. The great thing about this exercise is that it can be done anywhere—and I mean anywhere! If your day isn't going well, you can always take yourself off to the bathroom and sit there and focus on your breath until you can face the world again. It really helps to calm the mood and clear the mind. Even just three breathes like this can give you the power to transform your day.

If you like these short exercises and want more, jump over to the interactive version of the book and I will walk you through a few extra ways to de-stress.

l = love your liver and detox

There are many changes in menopause that can affect the functioning of the liver and contribute to the development of liver disease. The most common being fatty liver disease.

Estrogen exerts many liver-related benefits. It protects the liver by:
- inhibiting the formation and development of fibrosis (which can lead to a fatty liver)
- protecting against mitochondria damage (fatigue)
- inhibiting cellular senescence (where cells stop dividing and premature ageing occurs)
- increasing innate immunity (the ability to defend ourselves against toxic substances and bugs)

- promoting a favourable balance between an anti-oxidant and a pro-oxidant state (inflammation).

With the reduction of estrogen comes changes within the liver itself. Data has shown an approximate reduction in function at 1% per year starting in peri-menopause. Findings include:
- the reduction in liver blood flow and volume
- reduced overall function
- reduced ability to regenerate

In menopause, the main form of estrogen changes from estradiol (produced from the ovaries) to estrone (produced in the adipose tissue and liver). We need the liver to produce estrogen now but we also need estrogen for the proper functioning of the liver. Hence the increase in liver pathology at this time.

BUT your liver is amazingly resilient and in most cases, is capable of regeneration.

Before you start detoxing, it's a good idea to see how your liver is coping and what toxins it's finding challenging to remove. As mentioned in the investigate section, I recommended a blood test, appropriately called a liver function test or LFT, a urine test called GPL-Tox, to look for chemicals and a hair test, or Hair Tissue Mineral Analysis (HTMA), to discover if you are storing toxic metals.

It's not just toxins that can affect liver function, there are many viruses that compromise its function also. The first ones that spring to mind are the strains that cause hepatitis (A, B, C, D, E), but the herpes family of viruses (HSV1, HSV2, CMV, EBV, VV, HH6, HH7, HH8) can also cause liver damage. The rest of this section discusses generalised liver function and improvement, however if your underlying cause of liver dysfunction is viral related you will also need to reduce your viral load to see better longer-term results.

Signs and symptoms that your liver is overwhelmed and not optimally functioning include:

- Headaches
- Itchy skin
- Discomfort in your upper right quadrant (under the lower part of your ribs)
- Persistent fatigue and or weakness
- Nausea
- Easy bruising, easy bleeding and spider veins
- Swollen ankles, feet and belly
- Confusion and brain fog
- Skin pigmentation
- Insomnia
- Weight problems
- Constipation
- Chronic pain.

In order to start loving your liver, you first need to remove the number of toxic substances it's exposed to daily. You may want to go back and read the 'Nutritious foods' and 'Non-toxic environment' sections again.

The average woman is exposed to hundreds of chemicals every day, all of which her liver needs to process. A few easy changes like eating organic foods or changing your personal care products, allows the liver more breathing room. Less chemicals in, the less work the liver must do to remove them. Giving the liver breathing room allows it to go back and start processing the chemicals it has put into storage, as it was too busy to process them. The body can store chemicals almost anywhere. The liver prioritises getting toxins out of the bloodstream to prevent it getting to vital organs and potentially causing death. However, it still wreaks havoc in storage, e.g., lead loves your bones and it displaces calcium and makes your bones brittle.

If you discover during the testing phase that you have particularly high storage levels of a substance or substances, please seek individual care with a health professional. They can help you find your source of toxicity to prevent new exposures and then help you remove it. Removal can be problematic and time consuming. In general, it's better to go slowly and safely as you may feel very unwell detoxifying initially—but the renewal in health and vitality is worth it!

Foods that support optimal liver function:
- Globe artichoke
- Cruciferous vegetables like broccoli
- Spices: turmeric, garlic, ginger
- Citrus fruit: lemons
- Beetroot
- Protein: nuts, fish and eggs
- Greens: dandelion, coriander and spinach
- Berries: blueberries
- Avocado
- Spirulina
- Apple cider vinegar
- Water—it's essential to stay hydrated
- Herbal teas: milk thistle, dandelion, green tea.

Lifestyle practices work by stimulating lymphatic drainage. Anything that stimulates lymphatic movement encourages detoxification. Include as many of these lifestyle factors as possible:
- Dry skin brushing, towards the heart
- Any form of movement, such as walking, rebounding, yoga
- Stretching
- Massage
- Epsom salt bath.

e = exercise and other lifestyle factors

This section is probably the most important part of this book. Supplements are add-ons; they top up your results if you have a solid foundation. They may still help you lower your current symptom picture, however without addressing the following points, you have very little chance of any long-term success with staying symptom free.

These lifestyle habits are bricks that together build a solid foundation for long term success.

- Exercise
- Sleep
- Quitting Smoking.

Exercise is essential at every stage of life, and perimenopause/menopause is no exception.

Look at your current level of activity and see if it needs improving. I know that for some of you, I am preaching to the converted—and if this is you, well done and keep up the hard work. If this is not you, start from where you are. I have often seen that recruiting a friend or family member to join you and keep you accountable, is a good starting place. Book in times and days to get started. This may start with just a walk around the block and later extend to a full day hike in the mountains. It could start with a lap or two in the local pool or a short bike ride. You may even like to sign yourself up for a charity event, such as a fun run or walk-a-thon. Personally, this is where I started. I signed myself up for a 500 km charity bike ride, and I hadn't been on a bike for 20 years! Luckily, I had time to learn how to ride with gears (although I still do muck it up from time to time) and a deadline to get fit. I know this extreme approach doesn't work for everyone, but it did for me.

Ideally, you are looking for a combination of stretching, weights and cardio. It may be easiest to hire a personal trainer to help customise an individual program, get you started and keep you accountable. There is nothing like putting money on the table to get you moving and shaking. Exercise physiologists are a better bet if you have injuries or special needs. Exercise physiologists are both physiotherapists and personal trainers. If this is you, I would start with your GP and see if you can put together a care plan that includes exercise physiology. You may even be able to access these sessions on Medicare.

One of the most important aspects of exercise is fun. This is something you will have to do regularly, so find something you enjoy. Personally, I have found that if you find the right group, they will motivate or 'kindly bully' you into staying on track. Not that I endorse bullying, but sometimes a little tough love regarding getting moving and staying moving is needed— especially to help you get into shape.

Some of my favourite ways to exercise include:
- Walking, jogging or hiking
- Water sports such as swimming, aqua aerobics, surfing, kayaking, paddle boarding
- Cycling and spin classes (if you like to punish yourself)
- Bootcamp or Crossfit (but this isn't for the light-hearted)
- Dancing—all kinds
- Yoga, Pilates, Tai-chi
- Martial arts of any kind
- Team sports such as tennis, netball, soccer, softball or water polo.

Think about what team sports you enjoyed as a child as that can be the key to finding what you enjoy.

GET INSPIRED: THE BENEFITS OF EXERCISE
- It is one of the best stress management tools we have available.
- It helps balance out moods, is good at reducing depression and lifts moods in general.
- Regulates blood sugar levels. The more muscle mass you have, the more insulin receptors you have on your muscles. This means your body can regulate sugars better.
- Can improve your physical appearance by helping you lose weight and tone up
- Helps maintain bone mass and can help remineralise existing bone. It also strengthens cartilage, ligaments and muscles.
- Improves cognitive function. Exercise produces BDNF (brain-derived neurotrophic factor). BDNF has been shown to grow new brain cells! Yes, it is possible to grow new brain cells.
- Improves cardiac health by strengthening the muscles of your heart, improving the elasticity of blood vessels, increasing heart rate and blood flow.
- Better long-term energy production and increases oxygenation of your tissues.

- Your lungs get a workout as more oxygen gets flooded into your body.
- Reduces your risk of developing cancer (cancer hates lactic acid).
- Exercise can help delay the appearance of ageing skin. Thought that might get your attention, are you moving yet?
- Exercise can help improve your quality and quantity of sleep—in particular, morning exercise. If you exercise late at night, you may find your adrenaline levels are still raised post exercise and this may delay your sleep onset. If this is the case for you, exercise earlier in the day.
- Reduces your perception of pain and increases your pain tolerance.
- Finally, it can increase your sex drive.

Just a word of warning with exercise: don't overdo it! Excessive exercise can lead to increased adrenal stress, and we have already discussed the importance of keeping our adrenal glands happy. It can also increase your risk of injury.

In general, you need to move every day, but you don't need to work out every day.

Aim to workout at least 2.5 hours a week. You might go for a walk every day and three to four days a week include a class, weights session, swim or a bike ride. Make it fun. I love group classes because I love the energy in the room, but I also like a solo run. It's my escape from daily life; it's my meditation. So, commit, recruit some friends, or make new ones. Mix it up and have some fun.

SLEEP BETTER TO LIVE BETTER

There are many reasons for sleep issues at this stage of life and unfortunately, half of you won't sleep tonight. Stress and anxiety could be keeping your mind busy all night. Cortisol (a stress hormone) is usually involved in some shape or form with sleepless nights. Cortisol should peak around 7 am in the morning and drop during the afternoon, reaching its lowest point around 11 pm. If this level doesn't drop by the evening, sleep is almost impossible. Stress, worry and anxiety all increase cortisol levels. Cortisol increases blood sugar levels by converting stored glycogen into active blood sugar. Trying to sleep while stressed is like trying to sleep after drinking an energy drink filled with sugar—virtually impossible.

Melatonin is the hormone responsible for sleep. It works in opposition to cortisol. It starts to rise as the sun sets and drops as the sun rises. Hence, most of us could benefit from going to bed earlier and getting up earlier. Natural light exposure helps regulate it and unfortunately, blue light and other artificial light diminish it. Blue light is emitted from television screens, computers, tablets and phones. Some devices allow you to reduce the amount of blue light you are exposed to by using filters. There are also blue light blocking glasses. It's advised to avoid all screens 30-60 minutes before bed. It is also worth considering your household lighting. Consider investing in a lamp so you can reduce your general light exposure the closer it gets to bedtime.

Progesterone is a great sleep promoting hormone. Some of you during your fertile years might have noticed that it's harder to sleep just before your periods. If this was you, your body was responding to your dropping progesterone levels. For me, this was one of my first signs of perimenopause. As you get closer and closer to menopause, your progesterone levels get lower, and sleep may become a real struggle. Night sweats may also be waking you during the night.

Dietary factors like caffeine consumption and sugar can all contribute to a sleepless night. Alcohol may help you get to sleep but more often than not can give you a restless night.

A more serious possible reason behind sleep disturbances is sleep apnoea. Sleep apnoea affects over one million Australians. Sleep apnoea occurs when the walls of the throat come together during sleep and block off the upper airways. This leads to a halt in breathing until the brain recognises it lacks oxygen and signals to wake you up. Breathing then returns to normal as oxygen levels regulate. Many people with sleep apnoea snore loudly, as the body gasps for oxygen. Many people living with this condition have no idea they have it. Sleep apnoea is diagnosed with a sleep study. This can be done from the comfort of your bed. You will need to hire a polysomnogram. Check your local chemist to see if they rent these out. It's roughly AUD$100. A sleep study measures your blood oxygen levels, brain activity, heart rate and breathing. These results are uploaded from the machine and sent to a sleep doctor for a report and possible diagnosis. This report takes around five days. Alternatively, your GP can refer you to be tested in a sleep clinic. This will be significantly more expensive.

Health issues linked with the lack of sleep include:
- Increased weight.
- Lower moods and a higher tendency towards depression.
- Increased brain fog and cognitive decline (sleep is important for consolidation of memory). Sleep deprivation also increases amyloid plaque deposits by 25%, plaque build-up is a possible cause of Alzheimer's.
- Blood sugar disorders such as diabetes.
- Increased risk of cardiovascular disease (blood pressure).
- Decreased immunity.
- Hormonal disruptions.
- Increased stress levels and lower tolerance for stress.
- Increases the risk of any cause of death. Scary stuff!

LIFESTYLE FACTORS TO IMPROVE SLEEP
- **Timing.** Go to bed at a reasonable time every night. Set yourself a bedtime alarm if you need to.
- **Set the scene in your bedroom for intimacy and sleep only.** Remove the TV. Make sure the room is dark. Consider whether you need a new bed or pillow to help yourself feel more comfortable.

- **Be cool.** If being hot is keeping you awake, look at the tips for night sweats and bedding.
- **Environment.** Think about other aspects of the bedroom such as room temperature, noise, light and ventilation.
- **Turn off the tech.** Consider your bedrooms electro radiation field. Are you sleeping with your phone beside your bed? If you are, please move it or at least turn it onto flight mode at night. Moving it is a better option, that way you are not tempted to look at it. Is your modem nearby? If you use Wi-Fi in your home, please switch it off or put a timer on the device so it automatically switches off during your sleeping hours and switches back on when you're awake. It's also worth double checking your fuse box isn't on the other side of your bedhead.
- **Exercise.** Regular exercise can help physically tire you, so you are more likely to sleep.
- **Keep calm.** Deep breathing, prayer or meditation can help calm your mind before sleep.
- **Hot bath.** Try a hot bath before bed. Consider adding Epsom salts or lavender to enhance your relaxation.
- **Routine.** If you bring a baby home you need to teach it a sleep time routine, but do you have a routine? Now is the time to retrain yourself. It might be dinner followed by an evening stroll, hot bath, then into bed with a good book. Everyone is different—just see what works for you. I personally like the evening stroll, getting outside and away from artificial light, as it helps to increase your melatonin levels (sleep hormone). Dim your lights at home before you leave so your good work isn't undone by a blast of light as you get home.
- **Sunshine.** Try to spend some time in the sun every day. This helps to reset melatonin levels and therefore cortisol levels.
- **Weight.** Lose weight if you need to. Carrying extra weight increases your chances of sleep apnoea and worsening insomnia.
- **Reduce the blue.** Avoid blue light (light emitted from televisions and computer screens) before bed.

- **Coffee.** If you drink coffee make sure your last one was at least 8 hours before bed.
- **Music.** Play classical or other relaxing music to help unwind.
- **Tea time.** Drink herbal tea such as chamomile or a sleepy time blend.
- **Avoid drinking alcohol** before bed and of course, quit smoking if you're a smoker.

SUPPLEMENTS FOR SLEEP

- Magnesium: this is the relaxation nutrient, great for sleep, stress and muscle tension.
- B12 regulates sleep-wake cycles.
- L-Theanine: is a constituent in green tea that relaxes you. This can help if sleeplessness is due to stress, worry or a plain old busy head. Research has found it's also handy for improving cognitive function, emotional status, heart disease, obesity, cancer and even reducing the common cold.
- Melatonin: only homoeopathic melatonin is available over the counter in Australia. You will need a script from your GP to try it. It's great for resetting sleep patterns.

HERBS

- Black cohosh was found in a clinical trial to be a safe and effective way to improve sleep. It increased the duration of sleep and reduced the frequency of wakes during the night.
- California poppy works well if pain (especially nerve type pain) is keeping you awake. It is also useful for anxiety.
- Fennel is also clinically useful to improve sleep, hot flushes, vaginal dryness, vaginal itch and improve sexual satisfaction by reducing the discomfort/pain associated with dry intercourse.
- Lemon balm is a fantastic herb for women with a busy head, so it comes as no surprise that it is also found to improve sleep. I don't know about you, but most of my sleepless nights are due to my busy head, full of cyclic thoughts.

- Passionflower is a herb for anxiety and insomnia.
- Valerian: the research combines it with Lemon balm.
- Withania is also known as ashwaganda. This herb has been a personal saviour. It helps to take away your worries. It can reduce the amount of time it takes to get to sleep and improve the quality of your sleep.
- Zizyphus: can help to reduce the time it takes to get to sleep and increase total sleep time. It's also beneficial for brain health, memory and cognition.

There are two main types of insomnia. One is sleep latency or onset insomnia, this is where it takes an unusually long time to initiate sleep. The other is maintenance insomnia—where you wake regularly during the night. Some people have both.

If you struggle more with getting to sleep, initially consider trying:
- Magnesium
- Californian poppy
- Fennel
- Lemon balm
- Passionflower
- Valerian
- Withania
- Zizyphus.

Issues staying asleep once asleep:
- B12
- Black cohosh
- Withania.

QUITTING SMOKING

Smoking promotes earlier menopause. Smokers start having perimenopausal symptoms one to nine years earlier than non-smokers. The earlier you experience menopause, the more health risks you are exposed to later in life. They can also have more intense symptoms than non-smokers. Evidence suggests that this link is reversible and the earlier a woman quits, the less likely she is to be affected.

Smokers, in general, have lower estrogen levels. There are three suggested mechanisms for this:

1. Polycyclic hydrocarbons found in cigarettes can destroy ovarian germ cells and can cause premature ovarian failure.

2. Chemicals found in cigarettes such as nicotine prevent the conversion of androstenedione to estrogen.

3. Smoking disturbs the messaging from the brain to the ovaries via the hypothalamic-pituitary axis. It can delay the LH (luteinising hormone) surge, preventing ovulation and interrupting the menstrual cycle.

Smokers also have:

- Increased risk of breast cancer (by 19%).
- Increased risk of lung cancer (85% of all lung cancer is due to smoking).
- Increased risk of cardiovascular disease.
- Increased susceptibly to mood disorders such as stress, anxiety and depression.
- Increased risk of diabetes as it promotes insulin resistance and inflammation. In fact, smokers are 30-40% more likely to get Type 2 diabetes than non-smokers.
- Increased risk of premature ageing. Smoking can make your skin drier with less elasticity. Most smokers develop more wrinkles and more lines around their mouth, increased pigmentation, greyish skin tone, discoloured fingers and yellow teeth.

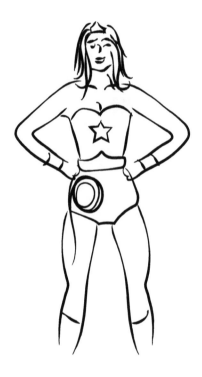

changes in menopause & what you can do about them

MENSTRUAL CHANGES

As discussed in the introduction, the first change is your body's ability to ovulate each month. With erratic ovulation comes reduced progesterone production. Your cycle length and bleeding may change. Spotting around menstruation can become commonplace. Nothing about your cycle is predictable anymore. Some women start to experience very heavy bleeds, others very light bleeds. Some cycles are very short and others very long.

Issues related to estrogen dominance such as endometriosis and fibroids can be exacerbated in early perimenopause due to the lack of opposing progesterone. Without a good ratio of progesterone, estrogen runs amuck. Estrogen is a growth hormone, which means it likes to grow a little fibroid here, a cyst over there and maybe a polyp as well.

Fibroids are common. It is estimated 60% of all women transiting into perimenopause have fibroids. The good news is that they usually self-resolve. But for a small group of women, they become so problematic in the early days that surgery is suggested. If you can survive through to post menopause, they shrink on their own—however the associated fibroid bleeding in perimenopause will annoy some women enough to get them removed.

Anaemia with heavy periods is common, and iron supplementation or infusions may be advisable. There are many herbal medicines that act as uterine astringents that can reduce blood flow. These herbal medicines include yarrow, lady's mantle, shepherd's purse or squaw vine.

HOT FLUSHES

Sorry gals, over 70% of you will experience hot flushes. The frequency can vary from every 30 minutes to once a week. The duration can last from a few seconds to half an hour. The good news is that for most of you, these will stop one to two years after menopause if left untreated. If treated however, they will resolve much faster, so start your supplements. Flushes are a mechanism of vasodilation (think red and hot) and tend to occur simultaneously with other symptoms such as sweating, palpitations, headaches, chills, fatigue, dizziness, nausea and difficulty concentrating.

Flushes may be due to estrogen decline and can be more severe in thin women, as fat stores can act as endocrine glands and also produce estrogen.

Stressed out women also seem to flush more as the adrenal gland is too overwhelmed to produce adequate amounts of estrogen. Instead, it produces noradrenaline. Noradrenaline is part of the sympathetic nervous system and helps to regulate body temperature. It regulates body temperature by narrowing the thermoneutral zone. If your temperature moves above the upper threshold of the thermoneutral zone you still start sweating. If it goes below the threshold you start shivering. So, the more stressed you are, the more noradrenalin you produce and the narrower your symptom-free zone is—which means the more prone to flushing and shivering you are. Hence the hot to cold movements in menopause: jacket on-jacket off syndrome. Noradrenaline is a flight or fight hormone. In the short term it can help you escape the Sabre-toothed tiger chasing you and live another day, but in the long term, it shuts down maintenance of your body and is linked with insomnia, loss of libido, digestive issues, lower resistance to infection, slower healing times, depression and addictions.

Enter serotonin. This neurotransmitter works in opposition to noradrenalin. It increases the thermoneutral zone and reduces hot flushes. It is also involved with regulating mood, digestion, sleep, memory and libido. I hope it's all starting to make sense now.

Estrogen increases serotonin levels and when estrogen drops, so does serotonin. This can increase most of the symptoms of menopause and not just temperature control. This is why antidepressant use seems to be all the rage in treating menopause these days. While I agree it is an option, it is not the first option in my opinion, as it has lots of possible side effects and it's very hard to wean off afterwards. Especially when there are other ways to increase serotonin levels with stress management techniques, such as exercise, massage, acupuncture, breathe work and meditation.

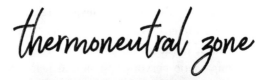

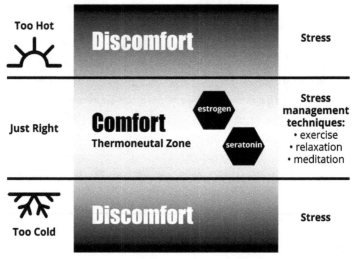

TRIGGERS FOR FLUSHES

These are not the same for everyone. You need to start making your list so you can avoid them or at least be prepared for the dreaded flush.

- Caffeine
- Alcohol
- Sugar and sugary or highly processed foods
- Allergenic foods such as gluten
- Spicy/chilli foods
- Stress, anxiety, fear, unresolved emotions, anger or even suppressed desires
- Heat, e.g., being on a train that isn't air conditioned on a hot day
- Exertion, e.g., running for your bus
- Smoking.

LIFESTYLE

Wear natural fibres that are light and loose fitting. Always layer your clothes so you can easily remove or add, depending on how you are feeling. There are many clothing ranges available that are especially designed to help keep you cool and reduce hot flushes. Here are a few:

- Cucumber clothing (https://www.cucumberclothing.com)
- Become (https://www.webecome.co.uk)
- Attune Womenswear (https://www.attunewomenswear. com).

It's also handy to have a handheld fan within reach.

Get adequate sleep. Research has shown that chronic sleep disturbances increase the frequency of moderate to severe flushing.

Try acupuncture, as it has had a long history of success and its results have been backed through research. My personal preference is Toyohari, the Japanese version of acupuncture.

Some women like to wear a wet towel across the back of their neck. Koldtec is a pimped up example of this. It's an ice towel. You simply freeze the inner ice strip and then insert it into the necktie when you want to wear it. It provides two hours of iced relief.

SOLUTIONS

- B complex: reduces your stress response.
- Vitamin C with Bioflavonoids: tones blood vessels and reduces vasodilation (hot flushes).
- Vitamin D: may reduce hot flushes by regulating serotonin levels.
- Vitamin E: reduces hot flushes as it alters the cellular response to estrogen. It also acts in a similar manner to progesterone.
- Omega 3 (sea buckthorn or fish oil): reduces frequency of hot flushes.

- Magnesium: regulates body temperature, vasodilation of blood vessels and helps reduce the stress response.
- Probiotics help to increase serotonin levels

HERBS

- Black Cohosh: phytoestrogenic, cooling and also good for hormonal mood changes.
- Motherwort: this herb is a great choice if the hot flushes are accompanied with palpitations, racing heartbeat and anxiety.
- Red Clover: hot flushes, night sweats, breast pain and anxiety.
- Rehmannia: a cooling herb that reduces flushing associated with stressful triggers.
- Sage: is the best herb for reducing excessive perspiration as it improves blood flow to the head and is estrogenic.
- Shatavari: this herb is specific for enhancing your libido. It also decreases dryness, hot flushes, night sweats, anxiety and stress.
- Tribulus: most successful herb in clinical trials for reducing hot flushes. It is also used for night sweats, libido, insomnia and sweating
- Zizyphus: reduces flushing associated with stress and/or anxiety. Can also improve sleep.

NIGHT SWEATS

Night sweats are simply hot flushes that occur at night and disturb your sleep. The same recommendations for hot flushes work here. For some women, they simply wake hot, for other women, they are so drenched that they sweat through their pyjamas and bedding as well.

If this is you, you may like to consider purchasing one of these:

- Cool Jams.[17] These pyjamas are softer and lighter than cotton and dry faster. Best of all they come with a 60-day money back guarantee. Love them or get your money back.

17. Cool-Jams, 2017.https://cool-jams.com.au

- Ooler Sleep System.[18] This actively manages the body's temperature overnight to deliver a magical deep sleep.
- There are many linen companies that specialise in cooler bedding. Easy Breezy sheets by Perfectlinens is one example.
- Nacreous Mattress Pad by Slumbercloud.[19] This temperature regulating mattress pad absorbs heat while you sleep.

Two things are certain: you must work on both reducing your flushes and improving your sleep patterns to see the best results.

Herbs to help your quality of sleep and reduce night sweats:
- Chamomile: relaxant, digestion, overall good bedtime herb
- Hops: specific for insomnia caused by flushing, can help regulate LH surges
- Oats: depression, exhaustion and insomnia
- Skullcap: insomnia and nervous tension
- Valerian: good if anxiety is keeping you awake
- Withania: improves sleep in general and relaxes the mind and body
- Zizyphus: specific for night sweats, insomnia and anxiety
- Melatonin specifically improves sleep.

SEXUAL HEALTH

'The better your sex life, the better your outlook.'
— Dr Berkson

Are you ready for some really good news?

World renowned psychosexual therapist, Dr Ruth Westheimer is 91 years young and recommends that we stay sexually active until the age of 99. If you are single, she recommends using a vibrator to help keep the vaginal tissue alive.

18. Ooler Sleep System https://www.chilitechnology.com
19. Slumber Cloud, 2019. https://www.slumbercloud.com/nacreous-mattress-pad.html

Regular sex promotes better memory and sharper focus. It's scientifically proven to increase grey matter and help prevent Alzheimer's. It also increases energy levels and improves mood.

Sex supplies more estrogen, oxytocin and testosterone to your brain. These hormones are fuel for your hippocampus. The hippocampus is all about memory (short and long term) and motivation. How cool is that? The more often you have sex, the better you think and the more motivated you are to get on with life!

Here are some tips from Dr Westheimer on sex as you age:
- Better times for sex are in the morning or early afternoon.
- Increase the amount of foreplay.
- Use lubricant (use pH balanced product like Yes WB[20]).
- All types of touch are important, so if you are single, have regular massages.
- Your orgasm is your responsibility.
- It's vital to have a healthy relationship above all. No one wants sex with someone they are not happy with.
- Try different positions! (She emphasises this).
- Sex is a time to go inwards, to forgot about the dishes and your to-do list and focus on connecting and enjoyment.
- Read erotic literature (she suggests *50 Shades of Grey*).
- Enjoy erotic art.
- Drink a little wine, but not too much. A little wine helps put you in the mood, a little too much reduces the function of your orgasms and makes you tired.
- Your orgasm may not be as intense as you age, but it can still be satisfying.
- Sex with your partner is not a sin or shameful. It is an essential part of your relationship.
- If you are having trouble in the bedroom, see a sex therapist.

20. The Yes Yes Company, 2019. https://www.yesyesyes.org

In Dr Berkson's book, *Sexy Brain*, she suggests that the more frequent your sexual encounters are, the lower your risk of hormonal cancers such as breast cancer. Preliminary research backs this theory.

Can you believe women (and men) who are sexually satisfied have statistically less plaque in their arteries? Well, the good news is this is what was indicated in the Women's Health Initiative medical research trial. This study involved 93,676 women and it also found older women had more sexual satisfaction than younger women.

Other benefits of sex discussed by Dr Berkson include:

• Increases immunity.
• Burns calories. Dr Berkson calls it 'intimacy cross-fit' as it also improves strength, flexibility, muscle tone and cardiovascular conditioning.
• Reduces stroke and heart attacks.
• Reduces stress.
• Improves sleep.
• Increases longevity and keeps you younger, longer.

VAGINAL HEALTH

As your estrogen levels start to decline so does your collagen production. One consequence of lower collagen is a thinning of the vaginal mucosa. This results in a drier, less elastic vaginal environment, which can lead to discomfort, itch, pain (especially with sex) and being more prone to infections and prolapses.

As we age, our vaginal pH also changes. It starts to rise and this changes the microbiome (the bacteria that lives there). A good vaginal pH is 3.6-4.5, but in menopause, it can rise to 7. Anything above 4.5 increases your risk of infections such as bacterial vaginosis and thrush. You can test your vaginal pH by buying some pH or litmus paper. Make sure you buy a variety that goes up in 0.5 increments. Start by placing this against the inside of your vaginal wall, wait a few seconds and compare the colour. If you have a high pH, it is recommended to start using special female probiotics pessaries. Wet the capsule and insert it into your vagina before bed. The general rule is to insert it in a cyclic manner. Most women do it seven nights in a month. The rest of the month you can take this orally.

LIFESTYLE SOLUTIONS

- What you don't use you lose; regular intercourse is highly recommended. If you are single, self-love is mandatory. One of my favourite doctors, Dr Christiane Northrup, recommends a minimum of three orgasms a week for all women transitioning into menopause and beyond. Not only does it help stimulate circulation to the area, but it also improves mental wellbeing. This being said, adequate lubrication is essential. Stop if you are experiencing pain. The best lubricants are Yes and Sylk, which are both free of nasty chemicals. Two other things to consider with lubricants are pH and osmolarity. If you use sex toys, you need to consider the type of material that is used in their manufacture.
- Pelvic floor exercises can be beneficial to strengthen this entire area and help prevent prolapses.
- Avoid vaginal douches, hygiene sprays and chemical-laden soaps.

NUTRITIONAL SOLUTIONS

- Probiotics: this can be taken orally or as a pessary.
- Vitamin A: can help repair tears in the mucous membranes.
- Vitamin C: is a crucial building block of collagen. It is also a good immune booster to prevent infections.
- Vitamin E: can be used as a pessary or an oral capsule. It reduces vaginal dryness and itching.

- Sea buckthorn: is a mucus membrane tonic, great for a dry vagina and/or dry skin. Fish oil can also work, but I find sea buckthorn is better for dryness. It can be taken as a pessary if vaginal dryness is the only issue. I generally recommend taking it orally to help with dry skin and full body lubrication.

HERBAL SOLUTIONS

- Fennel cream: topically applied fennel has been found to decrease vaginal itching, reduce dryness and improve sexual function and satisfaction, while reducing any discomfort with sex due to dryness.
- Tribulus: research has indicated this herb can help improve vaginal lubrication, increase genital sensations and the ability to reach an orgasm.

TESTING

- Vaginal litmus paper swab
- Pap smear
- High vaginal swab, including checking for ureaplasma, mycoplasma, and bacterial swab.
- Specialised do-it-yourself microbiome testing, such as Invivo Female Ecologix.[21]

BREAST HEALTH

As you approach perimenopause, you may start to notice changes in your breasts. Some women discover lumps and bumps, others notice changes in size or texture, new sensitivity or discomfort.

As your estrogen levels start to drop, you may notice your breasts start to shrink. This is because estrogen stimulates the glandular system for milk production. When you no longer need your breasts to be on standby for feeding, they may start

---

21. Invivo Female Ecologix, Microbiome testing,
    https://invivohealthcare.com/products/diagnostics/female-ecologix

to feel less dense, and this can lead to sagging. If you are a regular exerciser, especially if you use weights or do push ups, you might not notice this as much, as the exercise will increase and tone the muscles underneath to help keep your breasts up!

It's a good idea to do regular breast self-examinations. It's a better idea to ask your doctor to do an annual physical examination.

BREAST SELF-EXAMINATION

Start by getting comfortable with what 'normal' looks and feels like for you. Some women will have naturally lumpy breasts; other breasts may feel denser and more fibrous. It's normal to have a slightly different shape or size breast.

If you are still menstruating, breast self-examination is best to do a few days after your period ends.

1. Stand in front of a mirror with your arms relaxed by your side. Look at both breasts. Look for anything unusual. Check for skin dimpling or nipple pulling.

2. Repeat with your arms behind your head.

3. Repeat with hands on your hips. Bend slightly forward and pull your shoulders and elbows forward.

4. Squeeze each nipple and look for any discharge.

5. Lie on your back and put one arm over your head. With your other hand, start palpitating under your arm using an up-and-down pattern. Using the pads of your fingers feel for any abnormalities. Continue over the breast until your reach your sternum, then swap sides and repeat. To thoroughly check the entire area, make sure you feel up to your collarbone. Some women prefer to use circular or wedge-like patterns instead of lines. As long as the entire area is covered, it doesn't matter which technique you use.

examine yourself

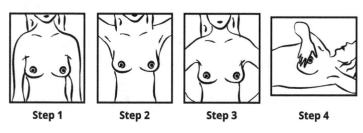

| Step 1 | Step 2 | Step 3 | Step 4 |

Here is a list of things to look for:
- A new lump in your breast or under your arm.
- Thickening or swelling of any part of your breast.
- Irritation or dimpling of your breast skin.
- Redness or flaky skin in your nipple area or your breast.
- Pulling in of your nipple, or pain in your nipple area.
- Persistent nipple itch.
- Nipple discharge.
- Any change in the size or the shape of your breast.
- Pain in any area of your breast.
- Warmth, redness or darkening of the skin around your breasts.

A medical doctor should investigate all new lumps and bumps and any new discomfort. Especially any sharp, shooting or radiating pain. Please note that nine out of ten lumps are not cancerous, but all are worth further investigation.

BREAST AUGMENTATION

I'm not a fan of implants. The risk to reward ratio in my opinion just isn't worth it. The most common complication is leaking and rupturing. Both cancer and autoimmune disease are linked with this. The increased risk of cancer that is linked with breast implants isn't actually breast cancer. It's a cancer of the immune system— Anaplastic large cell lymphoma.

If you have breast implants, know the longer you have them, the increased risk of rupture you will have. Another possible problem is the growth of mould or bacteria within the saline implants. If you are the kind of person that reacts to household mould you can start to imagine the extent of the damage the mould inside your body would have.

If you would like to know more watch the *Absolutely Safe* documentary or read *Breast Implants:Everything You Need To Know*, by Nancy Bruning.

DIET
Eat lots of the brassica family—broccoli, cabbage, brussel sprouts, cauliflower, etc.

LIFESTYLE
• Save your bras with underwire for special occasions and invest in everyday comfortable bras without underwire. It's best to get these fitted as most women are wearing the incorrect size bra and this increases discomfort.
• Switch to aluminium-free deodorants.
• Avoid cigarette smoke.
• Once you have had any uncomfortable lumps checked by a doctor, you may find relief by placing hot compresses over them.

TESTING
• Urinary iodine levels. Low iodine is a risk factor for breast changes such as fibrous or cystic breast.
• Physical examination by your doctor.
• Imaging can be ultrasound, mammogram or both. (Note, mammograms are contraindicated if you have breast implants as it can rupture the implants).

- If you are a Sydney based reader, I have some good news. St Vincent Clinic has one of the first 3D breast imaging machines. The test is called Abbreviated Breast MRI[22] and it is more accurate than mammogram and has obvious advantages: no breast compression and no radiation! Let's hope we get a few more machines spread through the country soon.

Note, I have specifically left out breast cancer treatment. If you have breast cancer, please do not self-treat. See a practitioner who specialises in the care of this form of cancer. It's your life, and you are worth it.

BONE HEALTH

Preventing osteoporosis should be a priority for all women. 90% of your peak bone mass is acquired by 18 years of age in females and continues to increase until the age of 30. Women start to lose about 1% a year until menopause and after menopause this increases to around 2-3% a year. This rapid increase in bone loss later in a woman's life is due to the decreasing levels of estrogen.

It is, therefore, easy to say that the better bone health you have in your earlier years, the easier it will be to have good bone health as you age. But all is not lost if you don't have great bones. Bones are alive, and bone cells are constantly renewing themselves, with your oldest bone cell being only 10 years old. It is possible to improve your bone health at any age in your life.

For the best bones possible, you need a combined approach of addressing your diet, supplements and lifestyle.

22. St Vincent's Clinic Medical Imaging & Nuclear Medicine, 2019. https://www.svcmi. com.au/abbreviated-breast-mri.html

DIET

The number one food you need for bone health is fat. Your bones have an outer fat layer—think of it as a fatty layer of mesh. This mesh gives your nutrients a place to attach and this strengthens your bones. Without this mesh, your nutrients can't help your bones, as they have nowhere to live. In your diet, you are looking at having seven to nine tablespoons of good fat a day. Good food sources include coconut, olive, nuts, seeds, avocado, eggs and seafood. I recommend taking oil supplements to ensure an adequate amount. In contrast, bad fats, think anything deep fried, partially hydrogenated fats (like those found in supermarket bought cakes and other baked goods), cottonseed oil, corn oil, vegetable oil, soybean oil, canola oil and trans fats, destroy bone health.

The second most important nutrient is protein. It strengthens your bone mesh and helps with bone regeneration or turnover. To get adequate protein, you need a protein source in every meal. Protein sources include fish, chicken, meat, eggs, cheese, tofu, nuts and seeds.

Foods to avoid include sugar and highly processed sugary food and drinks. Sugar is highly acidic, and it leaches calcium out of your bones to buffer the pH levels. This increases urinary excretion of calcium. This calcium is lost for good. It's also best to avoid gluten as it has been found to thin bones and increase inflammation.

Bones are a storage house of calcium for the heart, muscles, blood and nerves. If you do not have enough dissolved calcium in your blood, your body will take it from your bones. Having adequate calcium allows the body to redeposit the calcium in the bank (your bones). Try to consume non-dairy calcium sources. Dairy that has been pasteurised and homogenised has denatured the calcium in it, making it unable to be absorbed. Better calcium sources include seeds (especially sesame seeds), sardines, dark green leafy vegetables or nuts.

NUTRIENTS FOR BONE BUILDING

- **Vitamin A:** is a building block together with vitamin D for the production of connective tissue and the collagen matrix of cartilage and bone.
- **Vitamin C:** essential for bone repair and reduction of cortisol which is involved in bone breakdown.
- **Vitamin D:** activates alkaline phosphatase for bone remineralisation. It's needed to absorb and lock calcium into your bones enhancing bone remineralisation.
- **Vitamin K:** is involved in bone metabolism and the prevention of osteoporosis by activating osteocalcin which is a building block for the bone matrix. Food sources include spinach, silverbeet, broccoli, brussel sprouts, cabbage and lettuce.
- **Boron:** is essential in combination with calcium and magnesium for good bone maintenance. It also has a role to play in vitamin D activation.
- **Calcium:** best sources include citrate or malate. Avoid carbonate as it can increase your risk of kidney stones. High levels of calcium can cause bone spurs, kidney stones, bursitis, arteriosclerosis and glaucoma. It's no longer the solo golden supplement of bone health. Don't take this on its own. Having a combination product reduces your risk of complications.
- **Magnesium:** research is looking at the importance of magnesium over calcium for bone health. Magnesium helps keep calcium dissolved in the blood and stops it from being deposited elsewhere, such as in the kidney. Magnesium deficiency can contribute towards the development of kidney stones. Calcium on its own may be deposited in soft tissue rather than bone. Magnesium enhances bone building and remodelling.
- **Manganese:** is needed for skeletal and cartilage formation.
- **Potassium:** strengthens bones.
- **Resveratrol:** prevents bone loss.

- **Silica:** increases bone collagen and strengthens the connective tissue. It also increases the rate of bone mineralisation.
- **Zinc:** essential for collagen formation.

LIFESTYLE

- Exercise regularly with some kind of weight or resistance component. Ideally three to four times a week.
- See the sun. Don't burn but get outside and have some sunscreen-free exposure regularly.
- Excessive alcohol consumption robs bones of their health by slowing down bone reformation and accelerating bone breakdown.
- Cigarette smoking also accelerates bone breakdown. Stop smoking. Cigarettes contain cadmium which interferes with bone formation.
- Excess radiation exposure also weakens bone.
- Reduce stress due to the connection with cortisol and reduced bone mass.
- Lead accumulates over a lifetime and can get stored in your bones and teeth. These parts hold about 95% of the total body lead burden. As it's not stored in the blood, don't test for it in the blood. Blood tests for lead are only accurate during a recent lead exposure (usually within 28 days). As your exposure is more likely to have been decades ago, this isn't relevant. A hair test for lead is a better indication of stored lead levels. During your youth, having lead locked in your bones and teeth was a safer place to it store away. Unfortunately, during menopause when your bone mass is reducing, these stores can be mobilised. They leave their inert hiding place, re-circulate the body and re-enter the blood and soft tissue. High lead levels can cause an increase in blood pressure, an inability to sleep, concentration or memory issues, headaches and depression. It's important to get to the root cause of your symptoms so you can find a long term resolution. Thankfully for current generations, environmental lead levels are reducing these

days, but we grew up in the lead era. It was only removed from paint in 1978 so, it is possible to have lead-based paint and lead-based dust in older houses. It was removed from petrol in 2002.

Certain medications weaken bones. Please speak to your doctor if you are on any of these and are worried about your bone density.

- Corticosteroids (asthma, rheumatoid arthritis and other inflammatory conditions)
- Antacids
- Certain cancer medications such as Tamoxifen
- Some epilepsy medications
- Some antidepressants.

TESTING

- Dexa scan: to assess bone density
- HTMA: to check for metal toxicity such as lead and cadmium
- Vitamin D.
- PTH — parathyroid hormone: as it controls calcium levels
- Serum calcium: common manifestations of hypercalcemia include weakness and fatigue, depression, bone pain, muscle soreness (myalgias), decreased appetite, feelings of nausea and vomiting, constipation, polyuria, polydipsia, cognitive impairment, kidney stones and osteopenia or osteoporosis.

JOINT HEALTH

Osteoarthritis was once thought of as a disease of wear and tear alone. Today there is increasing evidence that estrogen influences the health of your joints and may be a contributing factor towards the development of osteoarthritis in at-risk individuals. It is thought that estrogen plays a role in the maintenance of articular tissues and of the joint itself, by reducing inflammatory cells from building up in the synovial fluid surrounding the joint. It's these inflammatory cells that start to damage the joint when they are left unchecked.

These are some of the other factors that will put you at a higher risk of joint issues:

- Being overweight: this increases joint wear and tear, especially the weight-bearing joints such as ankle, knees and hips.
- Having diabetes.
- Being inactive. The old saying 'use it or lose it' certainly fits here
- Overuse of isolated joints (RSI). We have all heard about tennis elbow.
- If you have ever been involved in a fall or accident that impacted certain joints.
- Certain infections are linked with joint breakdown such as staphylococcus aureus, streptococci and gonococci. Viruses such as Epsten Barr is also linked with joint issues.

If your joints are starting to flare, I highly recommend you find a team of local practitioners. I personally use a combination of chiropractic, acupuncture and massage however osteopathy, physiotherapy and exercise physiology could also be beneficial. I cannot emphasise the need for good and regular physical therapy. I still go when I'm not in pain because I want to maintain my feeling of wellness. Prevention is much better than a cure.

Diet plays a huge role in joint health. Beneficial fats found in seafood, eggs, coconut and olives all help lubricate the joint and prevent wear and tear. They are also anti-inflammatory which can help reduce the build-up of inflammatory, damage causing substances. Turmeric is another anti-inflammatory food which is fabulous for reducing joint pain. Unfortunately, it's poorly absorbed as a food substance so I would consider adding it as a supplement. This section wouldn't be complete without mentioning water. Dehydration exacerbates everything, including joint pain.

Supplements for joint health

- Fish oil especially ones higher in EPA for its anti-inflammatory qualities.
- Rosehip, natural vitamin C and GOPO are good for reducing joint inflammation.
- Anti-inflammatory herbs: turmeric, boswellia, ginger, cat's claw and devil's claw.
- Probiotics—yes, probiotics. There is research linking dysbiosis to joint pain.

MUSCULAR HEALTH

Many women complain about muscle pain whether it be cramping, spasms, twitches, general tension or even muscular fatigue or weakness. If you're not looking after your muscles, they won't look after you.

We have about 650 muscles in the human body and we need them to do anything and everything. There would be no smiling, chewing, breathing, beating heart, sitting up or walking without orchestrating the stimulation of several muscles at once. Muscles constantly work by contracting and relaxing—sometimes consciously, other times unconsciously. They need to be properly fuelled for optimal function.

Your body uses calcium for muscle contraction and magnesium for muscle relaxation. Most muscular issues are caused by the muscles inability to relax, e.g., a cramp, twitch, or spasm. Therefore, magnesium is one of the most useful minerals for happy muscles.

Potassium and sodium are other essential electrolytes for muscular health. They help regulate the flow of your muscular contraction.

Coenzyme Q10 is the first nutrient I think of for muscle weakness or muscle fatigue, especially if you are taking any heart medication. Many medications (especially statin-based ones) reduce your body's CoQ10 levels—which results in muscle issues and lower energy levels, amongst other things. CoQ10 is also preventative against muscular damage by reducing oxidative damage within your muscles.

Being iron deficient can also encourage the development of painful cramps. Iron deficient muscles don't have the energy to function as there is a reduction in both strength and stamina of the muscle.

Finally, vitamin D deficiency is linked with muscle pain and weakness. But this time it's more of a chronic issue.

NERVE HEALTH

Symptoms of poor nerve health include numbness, pins and needles, tingling, stabbing, throbbing, freezing, burning, weakness and sensitivity. The most common symptoms women complain about during menopause include the sensation of electric shocks, tingling extremities, burning tongue or burning feet.

Estrogen plays a role in being both neuroprotective and neurotrophic. This means it protects your nerves from damage and it also plays a role in growing new nerve cells. Hence, nerve issues are more commonly found in menopause—although there are plenty of other reasons why these symptoms can be occurring and it's important to first rule out other possibilities.

Type 2 diabetes is the most common cause of peripheral neuropathy. It is estimated 50% of people with diabetes will experience nerve pain, mostly commonly in the feet and legs.

Certain autoimmune diseases such as Multiple Sclerosis destroys nerve cells.

Other reasons include:
- Nutritional deficiencies, especially the B vitamin family (B1, B3, B6, B12).
- Previous injury.
- Excessive alcohol intake.
- Medications, such as cancer drugs.

- Certain viruses such as herpes, epstein barr and lymes.
- Exposure to heavy metals or other toxins.
- Systemic inflammation.

The very first item I address with nerve pain is B12. It's important B12 levels are at the very high end of the reference range—or even over the range—if you're experiencing nerve pain.

I often prescribe high-dose B12 injections. Alternatively, you can grab sublingual B12 lozenges and continually suck on them all day. B12 comes in four forms, but methylcobalamin is my preferred form for nerve issues.

B12 is essential for building and maintaining your myelin sheath over your nerves. The myelin sheath is the insulating cover over your nerves that allows for conductivity. B12 also increases the speed of the messages that are sent along your nerves.

My second favourite supplement with nerve pain is alpha lipoic acid. Actually, it's the specific treatment option if the nerve pain is diabetic related. Alpha lipoic acid is a very strong antioxidant and is ideal for nerve issues as it crosses the blood-brain barrier.

Other useful supplements include:
- Fish oil, for its anti-inflammatory benefits.
- Magnesium, to relax the muscles around the nerves.
- Vitamin D deficiency is an independent risk factor for the development of peripheral neuropathy.
- Acetyl l carnitine is neuroprotective and antinociceptive. This means not only does it protect the nerve it also helps to block the detection of a painful stimulus by sensory neurons—meaning it reduces pain.
- Phosphatidylserine: supports the protection of healthy nerve cell membranes and can slow down the progression of nerve damage.

Additional strategies include:
- Chiropractic or osteopathic treatment is a must.
- Acupuncture can also be effective.

DIGESTIVE ISSUES

If you want to age well, live well and experience true health, you must have an optimally functioning digestive system! Don't underestimate the importance of good digestion and don't overlook treating it first and foremost.

Once your diet is cleaned up, most women find that their digestive function improves, and the microbial balance restores. You may discover a whole new level of health and vitality. This isn't surprising when you realise your digestive system is responsible for and linked with so many aspects of your health.

As we age, our body reduces its production of digestive enzymes and digestive acids. This means our ability to correctly breakdown food reduces, and symptoms can start to appear. Foods that you used to be able to eat without concern are now making you feel sick. Food sensitivities, bloating, gas, heartburn, altered bowel movements, cramps and haemorrhoids are becoming more common. If you find yourself minimising or avoiding animal products because you can't digest them, you need to re-ignite your digestive fire. Avoiding protein only makes this problem worse and creates new problems like zinc, iron or B12 deficiency. You actually need more protein, not less as you age. A low protein diet increases the rate of age-related skeletal muscle re-modelling. Ageing muscles have a lower percentage of muscle tissue and higher amount of fat cells. You don't want to accelerate this process.

Our good bacteria, the probiotics that make up our microbiome, may have been removed over a lifetime of antibiotic use, alcohol consumption or poor diet choices. Replacing them is vitally important. The health of your microbiome directly impacts all aspects of your health and happiness. If you don't have the right strains in the right places, it's too easy for pathogenic (bad) bugs to take over. Consider having a microbiome test. This detects beneficial and pathogenic microorganisms in the digestive system.

The quality and quantity of food we consume is also an issue. Standard farming practices are reducing the amount of nutrition in our food and adding toxins like glyphosate to our plate.

It's time to get back to a good old-fashioned clean diet. See the 'Nutritious foods' section for more details.

Signs your digestive system isn't working well

- Nutritional deficiencies such as vitamin B12, are generally an indication that your digestive system is struggling and it could be that it lacks the digestive fire to break down the food and release the nutrients. Or, it could be an issue with the digestive lining not properly absorbing the nutrients.

- Recurrent infections. Your digestive system is the first line of attack against invading pathogens. The stomach's acidic condition is designed to kill infections on contact. An imbalanced microbiota further down the digestive tract also causes immune dysfunction.

- Issues with mood, such as anxiety and depression. Your digestive system houses over 80% of your neurotransmitters. Have you heard of the gut-brain axis? We used to think most of the neurotransmitters that control your mood were contained in your brain—but we were wrong. It's actually your gut microbes that produce most of your neurotransmitters.

- Skin problems can be caused by dysbiosis, an imbalance in your gut microbes. Staphylococcus has been shown to trigger eczema, SIBO or small intestinal bacterial overgrowth which is linked with rosacea. Candida overgrowth can be linked with psoriasis and issues digesting gluten can be the cause of dermatitis herpetiformis.

- Memory and cognition issues can be linked with any food sensitivities. Have you ever experienced brain fog after eating a meal? Undiagnosed or poorly managed Coeliac's disease (gluten allergy) is strongly correlated with Alzheimer's disease.

- Research links poor digestion with poor sleep, but this is also true in reverse—poor sleep can exacerbate poor digestion. It's the case of 'what came first the chicken or the egg?'. Always start addressing the gut first.

- Dysbiosis increases inflammation and reduces your pain tolerance.

- Weight issues with either losing or gaining too much weight have been linked to an imbalanced microbiota.

- Poor digestion and food sensitivities can cause headaches and migraines.

- Hormonal imbalances. Have you heard of the Gut-Hormone connection? Estrobolome is a collection of digestive microbes that regulate the circulation and excretion of estrogen. They do this by producing beta-glucuronidase, an enzyme that activates estrogen. Too much or too little of this directly impacts on your hormone levels.

- The presence of an autoimmune disease can often indicate your digestive system isn't functioning optimally.

- Increased intestinal permeability, otherwise called leaky gut, can allow food particulars that are usually too large to be absorbed, to be absorbed, which can trigger allergic reactions.

- Certain food allergies can trigger asthma, sinus and other breathing issues. Common foods that may cause breathing problems include dairy, wheat, eggs, peanuts, soy and seafood.

- One of the most common complaints associated with poor digestion is fatigue. Think about Christmas afternoon, when you have eaten far too much food and all you want is an afternoon nap. Some people feel like this every day, as their digestive systems are overburdened and can't work optimally. These people need a major diet overhaul and lots of gut healing work.

- Small intestinal bacterial overgrowth (SIBO) is linked with coronary artery disease (CAD), which researchers call the Gut-Heart connection. The only problem is, researchers can't tell if SIBO causes CAD or if CAD causes SIBO. Maybe it's a two-way street as SIBO increases the production of bacterial by-products which may predispose a person to CAD, and CAD produces pro-inflammatory cytokines that lead to changes in the digestive microbiome.

Food as medicine

Apple cider vinegar. A tablespoon in a glass of warm water before meals can help increase your digestive ability and reduce heartburn, bloating, wind and constipation.

Fresh lemon juice. I use half a lemon squeezed in a glass of room temperature water and drink this as part of my morning routine.

Pineapple and pawpaw naturally contain digestive enzymes so eat them when they are in season.

These herbal teas soothe the digestive system: peppermint, chamomile, dandelion, ginger, marshmallow tea and fennel.

Stewed apple with cinnamon. Here's a delicious recipe that improves digestion, mucosal repair and is a food source for your good probiotics (prebiotic). It also boosts immunity, decreases inflammation and improves mood and energy levels. The perfect functional food!

RECIPE

- Take 6 granny smith apples and peel them.
- Add half a cup of water and 2 teaspoons of cinnamon.
- Simmer for 15 minutes and then set aside to cool.
- Divide into 4 servings. (It can be refrigerated for later consumption)
- Add probiotics when serving.

Important supplements:

- Slippery elm powder. This can be purchased at a health food store as either a powder or capsule. The powder is mixed with water to make a gravy-like consistency that you need to drink quickly and follow it up with a large glass of water. Slippery elm can help regulate bowel movements and ease heartburn as it coats, soothes, protects and heals your mucous membranes. Warning: if you are taking supplements it can reduce the absorption of these, so take them at different times.
- Digestive stimulant containing HCL and enzymes, to help digest your food.
- Multi-strain probiotic formula, to help restore the balance of good bacteria.
- Digestive repair formula containing glutamine and zinc, smooths and repairs the mucous membrane lining of your digestive tract.

Testing
- Comprehensive stool analysis
- Food allergy testing
- Microbiome testing.

FATIGUE

We have all had one of those days when you don't want to get out of bed, drag your feet all day and can't wait to get back to bed as soon as possible. If this describes you more often than a random day here and there, then read on.

There are many reasons for fatigue:
- Low hormone levels
- Mitochondrial dysfunction
- Insomnia/sleep apnoea
- Sugar imbalances
- Vitamin B12 deficiency

- Iron deficiency
- Vitamin D deficiency
- Toxicity (toxic metals, chemicals)
- Infections
- Liver issues
- Thyroid dysfunction
- Depression, stress, prolonged anxiety
- Respiratory disease
- Heart disease
- Adrenal fatigue.

One of the biggest causes of fatigue is mitochondrial dysfunction. Think of your mitochondria as the batteries in your cells that provide your power. If they are out of charge, so are you! Technically they produce energy by the process of oxidative phosphorylation where nutrients are converted into adenosine triphosphate (ATP). Unfortunately, the DNA in your mitochondria is very prone to damage. This damage results from external mechanisms such as environmental or pharmacological toxins and internal mechanisms such as being exposed to reactive oxygen species. Common signs of mitochondrial damage include fatigue, pain, weakness, and depression. Mitochondrial fatigue is not relieved by rest. Heads-up, this is one the rare times I don't test, as the best way to test for mitochondrial dysfunction is with a muscle biopsy. I find clinical signs are just as useful and less painful!

My favourite mitochondrial kickstart nutrients include:
- Acetyl l carnitine, this is a fat transporter, it transports the fuel into the mitochondria to be burnt as energy.
- Alpha-lipoic acid, especially if there are blood sugar issues alongside the fatigue.
- Antioxidants like Vitamin E and Manganese. Manganese is the primary anti-oxidant found in the mitochondria. It is essential for the protection against and removal of reactive

oxygen species.
- B vitamins – especially B2 and B3
- CoQ10 – but I prefer the ubiquinol form
- Glutathione or glutathione building blocks like selenium and N Acetyl Cysteine (NAC)
- Magnesium – as low intercellular magnesium is linked with mitochondrial damage

If you have a history of Epstein Barr Virus (EBV) it is also worth considering supplements such as L-lysine to reduce your viral load. EBV is a well-known mitochondrial damager and is linked with the development of Chronic Fatigue Syndrome.

Depression, stress and prolonged anxiety are also causes of fatigue.

Respiratory and cardiovascular disease both cause fatigue. Improving the underlying disease will help increase your energy level.

Lifestyle considerations to improve your energy include:
- Optimising your mindset. Low moods cause low energy levels. Start making changes in your outlook on life. Women with positive attitudes, who live with passion and purpose live longer, happier and more energetic lives.
- Think about what is dragging you down. What is taking your energy? Is it a bad relationship? Is it a toxic job? Stop giving your energy away. Making hard choices in the short term will provide you with a new lease on life and abundant energy in the long term.
- Being in a space of gratitude, will help renew your energy levels.
- Meditation, breathing exercises and mindfulness are essential habits you must cultivate in order to restore your vitality.

- Exercise is a non-negotiable. You need to move, this stimulates blood and lymphatic flow, and gets your oxygen and nutrients moving into your cells. It's the amount of exercise that can be a problem. If you are very fatigued it may just be a walk around your home, I would prefer a walk outside in nature but you need to start where you are, and build as you are ready, as overdoing it can be very fatigue-producing indeed.

Consider your environment. Fatigue is the #1 symptom of a toxic environment. Is your home filled with mould? How many toxic substances are in your kitchen, bathroom or garage? It's time to ditch them and find chemical-free alternatives. Have you ever tested your electromagnetic field (EMF)? Is your Wifi on 24/7? Are you zapping yourself and your cells? There is scary research linking EMF to mitochondria damage. Go back and reread the non-toxic environment chapters if needed.

Nutrition for energy
Ditch the sugar and stimulants. I understand that you might be currently using these as a crutch to get through the day, but ultimately, they have to go!

Add to this list the removal of processed, deep-fried, food-like substances.

It's time for a fresh approach. Lots of vegetables and salads, some fruit, good quality animal protein, and beneficial fats. It goes without saying that I recommend that these are all organic.

I find herbal medicine to be a powerful addition to help overcome fatigue. Some of my favourite energy restorative herbs include:

- Rhodiola, especially in the case of high stress.
- Withania, good for nervous exhaustion.
- Ginseng family: Korean, Siberian, American.

- Rehmannia combines well with licorice to help restore the adrenal glands.
- Echinacea: great if you are run down, tired or prone to catching infections.

COGNITION AND MEMORY

Regardless of whether you are working in a high-pressure job or enjoying retired life, most of us could do with a little more brain power.

The brain has many enemies, the two main molecules to watch out for are beta-amyloid plaque and tau tangles.

Beta-amyloid is produced and eliminated in the brain every day (released when synapses fire between nerve cells). The trouble comes however, when the brain accumulates too much beta-amyloid or can't eliminate it fast enough and it starts to clump together. These clumps are called beta-amyloid plaques. These plagues prevent messages from being sent across the synapses and causes neuron (brain cell) death.

Tau tangles are also a part of normal everyday brain function. They can help smooth the way for the transmission of signals along the axons and dendrites (these are protrusions that connect the networks of neurons together). Under certain conditions these can accumulate and become misshaped and toxic, causing messages to get lost in the brain and communication pathways to be shut off, inflamed or die prematurely.

I love the book by Jean Carter, *100 Simple Things You Can Do to Prevent Alzheimer's and Age-Related Memory Loss*. I have included some of her suggestions below, but I highly recommend you read her book if this area is of interest to you.

Foods to help improve cognition

- **Increase antioxidant-rich foods.** These foods reduce cognitive decline and prevent oxidation. The brain is the primary target of free radical damage. Eating at least three serves daily will help slow down the rate of cognitive decline by 40%. The best sources are:

- » Fruit: all types of berries, plums, cherries, apples, pears, oranges
- » Vegetables: artichoke, garlic, red cabbage, red leaf lettuce, leafy greens, asparagus, sweet potato, broccoli, brussel sprouts, kale, cauliflower, beetroot, radishes and spinach.
- **Alcohol.** Moderate drinkers (which means one drink for females, two drinks for males a day) have a 37% reduced risk of Alzheimer's than non-drinkers. Drinking more than this doubles the risk. Heavy drinkers account for more than 10% of all dementia cases.
- **Eat a choline rich diet.** Choline prevents memory decline by reducing inflammation and homocysteine levels in your brain. Choline rich foods include eggs, pistachios, cashews, almonds, shrimp, fish, meat, spinach, cauliflower and brussel sprouts.
- **Add cinnamon.** Cinnamon reactivates insulin and decreases insulin resistance. It also blocks and destroys the formation of filaments associated with Alzheimer's.
- **Enjoy dark chocolate.** High cocoa-containing products contain the antioxidant flavanol. Flavanol increases blood flow to the brain which stimulates regeneration of nerve cells and enhances the production of new ones.
- **Eat curry.** Indians have the world's lowest rate of Alzheimer's. Researchers put this down to the amount of turmeric consumed in their daily diet. Turmeric acts as an anti-inflammatory and antioxidant agent as it blocks the build-up of amyloid plaques and disintegrates current plagues. Eat yellow curries, as red and green do not contain turmeric.
- **Increase foods that contain B3 (niacin)** as they prolong the life of brain cells. Food sources include tuna, chicken, turkey, salmon and sardines.
- **Eat nuts.** Walnuts contain brain protective antioxidants. Research suggests eating seven to nine walnuts daily reduced oxidant damage to brain cells, reduced inflammation, stimulated new neuron (brain cell) growth and promoted

communication between existing cells. It also improved the general structure of the brain by blocking and removing beta-amyloid plaques.

- **Use olive oil.** It's an antioxidant and stabilises the membranes of brain cells. It contains a compound called oleocanthal which prevents the production of beta-amyloid plaques and prevents existing plagues from attaching to nerve cell synapses. Do not cook with it but instead drizzle over food before eating.
- **Drink tea, especially green tea.** Tea has been shown to reduce cognitive loss by blocking beta-amyloid plaque production and chelating and removing excess iron from your brain.

Reduce these foods to save your brain

- **Balance your blood sugar levels.** Alzheimer's has also been called 'diabetes of the brain' or Type 3 diabetes. High blood sugar levels and insulin resistance cause death to your delicate brain cells. A low-sugar diet can drop levels of beta-amyloid by 25%.
- **Reduce carbohydrates, especially grains.** Low carb diets result in less beta amyloid deposits. Giving them a greater than 50% reduced risk of Alzheimer's.
- **Avoid Gluten.** There is a very strong link between undiagnosed Coeliac disease and Alzheimer's. A gluten-free diet in these cases often reverses the cognitive dysfunction. If you or a loved one are having cognitive issues and digestive issues its best to test for Coeliac's disease. In the past, Coeliac's was thought of as a childhood condition. These days the number of adults being diagnosed is dramatically on the increase.
- **Avoid bad fats.** As they can increase the risk of Alzheimer's by four times. These fats strangle brain cells, stiffen and shrivel membranes, stunt dendritic cells, dry up neurotransmitters (which are needed for memory storage) and increase toxic beta-amyloid plaques.

- Avoid processed meats containing nitrosamines (e.g., cured meats, hams, hot dogs, bacon, salami). Nitrosamines damage your brain and reduce your cognition.

Lifestyle techniques to enhance your brain's capability

- **Be social.** Being social signifies an all-round better cognitive ability.
- **Get enough sleep.** Sleep deprivation increases beta-amyloid plaque by 25%.
- **Keep balanced.** Decline in physical balance is one of the first signs of future dementia. Good balance equals a three times reduced risk of cognitive issues. If you can stand on one leg for greater than 30 seconds with eyes open and arms crossed over the chest, that's good. If you can't do this, chiropractic treatment may help.
- **Exercise.** Exercise increases BDNF (brain-derived neurotrophic factor) otherwise known as 'the master molecule of the learning process'. It stimulates the growth and survival of new brain cells. BDNF naturally reduces as we age causing a reduction in memory and cognition. Exercise increases brain function in general by improving blood flow to the brain and promotes the production of new brain cells. The best type of exercise to improve cognitive function is aerobic exercise, combined with resistance exercise. One hour three times per week or half-an-hour, five times per week is ideal.
- **Play games.** Keep mentally active. Remember if you don't use it, you lose it. Play card games, do crossword puzzles, play board games or play computer brain games.
- **Join a book club or start a writing course.** Reading, writing and stimulating group discussion are all powerful ways to boost your brain function.
- **Meditate.** People who meditate regularly tend to retain more grey matter in their brain. This has been shown to help sustain attention and lessen cognitive decline as they age.

- **Increase self-esteem.** Women with higher self-esteem and more control over their lives have been shown to have less cognitive issues.
- **Have self-discipline.** Being goal-directed, dependable, careful, precise, orderly and detail-oriented means you are less likely to develop Alzheimer's.
- **Maintain your heart health.** High blood pressure has been implicated in cognitive defects later in life.
- **Seek help for depression.** Depression can be both a cause and symptom of cognitive dysfunction. Fretting, getting upset, being stressed out or in a low mood may also damage an ageing brain.
- **Get a higher education.** It's never too late to start. Studying encourages concentration, focus and reading stimulates brain cells to build better connections, which over a lifetime can prevent against cognitive decline.
- **Avoid environmental toxins.** Chronic exposure to environmental toxins can increase the risk of age-related memory impairments. If you have been exposed to these toxins, get a hair tissue mineral analysis and GPL-TOX panel to detect how high your levels are, and which toxins are in the highest concentration.
- **Check your eyes.** Untreated poor vision is a strong predictor of dementia. Beta-amyloid plaques can show up as unusual cataracts. The degree of cell death in the retina, mimics that in the brain.
- **Google something.** Surfing the net exercises your brain. It is a demanding exercise that forces you to make multiple decisions as you click through. This constant decision making engages essential cognitive circuits in your brain. Mental activity, like physical activity, strengthens your brain.
- **Reduce cold sores.** There is a correlation between cold sore outbreaks on the face and increased beta-amyloid plaque build-up in the brain. If you suffer with cold sores, take action

to reduce the incidents of outbreaks. L-lysine and zinc are a good start.

- **Learn a second or third language.** Handling more than one language constantly exercises the brain and helps counter dementia in later life.
- **Get out in nature.** Interacting with nature has similar effects on the brain as meditating; that is, increased attention and better short-term memory.
- **Do something new.** Having new experiences stimulates dendrite growth in nerve cells and therefore expands the brain's volume.
- **Switch off the TV.** Television viewing is the most dangerous leisure activity we have in our modern society. It switches off your brain. For every hour a day you watch TV, your risk of Alzheimer's jumps by 30%.
- **Be in the healthy weight range.** Excess weight shrinks your brain and makes it more vulnerable to cognitive decline.
- **Treat sleep apnoea.** During an acute apnoea episode, brain vessels constrict, starving nerve cells of oxygen, causing them to die and the brain to shrink. This process triggers extra inflammation and further neuron death.
- **Quit smoking.** It doubles your risk of cognitive issues.

Supplements for brain health

- **Antioxidant combinations.** Nutrients like alpha lipoic acid and acetyl-l-carnitine are strong antioxidant rejuvenators of ageing brain cells. They help prevent brain damage.
- **B vitamins.** B3 prevents memory failure by preventing and removing tau tangles. It also strengthens cellular scaffolding that carries information and prolongs neuron life. B6 has been found to boost memory. B9 reduces age-related damage and increases the brain's ability to self-repair. It also reduces homocysteine (a blood factor that damages the DNA of brain cells). B12 deficiency shrinks your brain

by breaking apart the myelin sheath (a fatty protective layer around the nerves). It also increases homocysteine and triggers inflammation. Symptoms can include brain fog, confusion, personality changes, mood swings and loss of balance.

- **Fish oil (especially the DHA component)** prevents blood clots, reduces inflammation, builds bigger neurons with stronger connections, slows the ageing process by lengthening telomeres, and destroys beta-amyloid plaque deposits and tau tangles.
- **Multi-vitamin** takers were found to have longer telomeres (telomeres indicate how fast a person is ageing biologically). It's best to get a high antioxidant formula with increased levels of resveratrol, vitamin C, E, and minerals selenium and zinc.
- **Phosphatidylserine** feeds the brain and improves cognitive abilities, enhances focus and helps retain information.
- **Phosphatidylcholine** boosts cognition, energy, builds healthy cell membranes, muscle recovery, aids in liver repair, improves digestion and may reduce cholesterol levels.
- **Herbal medicine.** Ginkgo, brahmi, rosemary, and gotu kola are all effective cognitive enhancers.
- **AVOID** copper and iron supplements (unless proven necessary by blood tests), as excess copper slows the brain's ability to remove amyloid plaques and excess iron causes inflammation of the brain and increases neurodegeneration (degeneration of the brain).

Useful tests

- The gene test for Alzheimer's is APOE4. People with this gene are more likely to get the disease earlier and more severely. However not everyone with this gene develops Alzheimer's. If you have it, make a conscious effort to make as many of the changes as possible.
- Blood sugar and insulin levels.

- Coeliac disease (anti-gliadin and tissue transglutaminase). The downside of this test is that you need to be eating gluten for it to be accurate.
- Blood Pressure.
- Homocysteine. High homocysteine predicts age-related memory loss, dementia and Alzheimer's. It's also an indication, you are not correctly methylating your B vitamins.
- Thyroid function test. Hyperthyroid kills neurons, depletes acetylcholine and damages cerebral blood vessels. Hypothyroid increases beta amyloid plaques.
- Copper.
- Iron and ferritin.
- B12.
- Vitamin D. Low vitamin D increases your chances of dementia by 394%! It works via the immune system by encouraging macrophages to remove beta amyloid plaques.
- HTMA (hair tissue mineral analysis for heavy metals).
- Sleep apnoea.
- Eye check-up.
- Dental check-up. Tooth and gum disease has been linked with memory issue.

HEART HEALTH

The current leading cause of death for women is heart disease. Most heart disease is lifestyle related. Now is the best time to start reducing your cardiovascular risk factors as lifestyle diseases are preventable and often reversible.

Risk factors for heart disease include:
- Being a smoker.
- Being overweight.
- Not regularly exercising.
- Having long-term stress or anxiety.

- Having blood sugar irregularities such as insulin resistance or diabetes.
- Genetics such as MTHFR. Having MTHFR alone doesn't hurt you, it's the lifestyle factors such as liver toxicity and poor diet with low folate containing vegetables that switch this gene on.
- High homocysteine, which can be due to MTHFR and low B vitamins especially B12.
- High cholesterol, high triglycerides, high LDL, low HDL, high lipoprotein A—all of which can be diet related.
- Having high blood pressure. This can be weight-related, stress related or nutritionally related.
- Having poor dental hygiene.
- Nutritional imbalances, e.g., high ferritin (iron) or sodium, low magnesium or potassium.

Solutions

- Vitamin C helps regulate blood pressure and cholesterol.
- Vitamin D deficiency may be linked with heart disease, stroke, heart attack and dangerous cholesterol levels.
- Vitamin E may reduce total cholesterol and LDL's (low-density lipoprotein)
- Fish oil can lower blood triglycerides.
- Resveratrol lowers LDL cholesterol and has an anti-platelet effect.
- K2 reduces artery calcification and plaque.
- B12 lowers homocysteine.
- B9 may lower blood pressure.
- Calcium is needed for muscular contraction and works opposite to magnesium. Together they regulate electrical conduction and blood pressure.
- Magnesium is a muscle relaxant. As your heart is made up of cardiac muscle fibres, and your blood vessels are filled with smooth muscle, magnesium is needed for their ability to

relax following a contraction. Magnesium also helps stabilise electrical conduction and is a vasodilator

- CoQ10. This antioxidant is reduced if taking cholesterol medication. It can improve oxygenation levels, energy levels, may reduce LDL and lower blood pressure.

Herbs

- Hawthorn is the most respected herb for heart health. It's best known for its ability to tone the heart and reduce blood pressure.
- Ginkgo improves circulation.
- Motherwort is the herb of choice for women experiencing palpitations with their hot flushes.
- Withania is a relaxant. It slows down thought patterns and reduces blood pressure.

Testing

- BP
- Cholesterol, triglycerides, LDL, HDL, Lipoprotein A
- MTHFR
- Fasting homocysteine
- Ferritin
- Fasting glucose, insulin and HbA1c
- Vitamin B12.

URINARY TRACT DYSFUNCTION

INCONTINENCE AND URINARY FREQUENCY

A woman's urinary health can start to deteriorate with menopause. The official name is urogenital atrophy. While this term includes the vagina as well as the urinary tract, we are going to focus on the urinary system here. Atrophy means to deteriorate or the wasting away of muscles. Common symptoms include the need to urinate more frequently, incontinence (or the inability to control urination) and being prone to urinary tract infections. We will discuss infections in the next section.

The main cause of urogenital atrophy is the lack of estrogen. As estrogen levels reduce, the bladder starts to weaken as does the urethra (the tube that carries urine out of the body), reducing your ability to control urinary function.

Another cause of urinary dysfunction is pelvic prolapse. Here, organs of the pelvic area drop into the vagina. This is due to the trauma of vaginal childbirth and the weakening of pelvic muscles due to the reduction of estrogen. Pelvic organ prolapse weakens the pelvic floor muscles, and this results in urge incontinence (frequent, sudden, strong urges to urinate, with the possibility of not making it to the bathroom in time) or painful urination.

Do you know there are specifically trained physiotherapists called pelvic physios? They focus on the health of a women's pelvic region. If you are struggling with urinary dysfunction, this is where I would start. They will investigate you for prolapse and design an exercise program to help you strengthen your pelvic floor muscles. They can also see if you are a suitable candidate for:

- Biofeedback therapy. This technology helps retrain your pelvic floor muscles and increases the amount of urine your bladder can hold plus helps control the timing of urination.
- Electrical stimulation of the bladder muscles—another possible treatment path.
- Vaginal pessary ring. This device is inserted into the vagina to help it hold up a prolapsed bladder.
- Urethral insert. This is a small tampon-like disposable device that is inserted into the urethra before a specific action such as exercise, that could normally trigger incontinence. This acts as a plug and needs to be removed before you next urinate.
- Surgery. There are various surgical techniques they can look at if you are not improving.

Acupuncture could also be beneficial.

If you don't currently have urinary symptoms but want to reduce your risk of developing them, daily general pelvic floor exercises can help. If you have never done these before, the easiest way to isolate these muscles is on the toilet. Start a urine flow and then stop it, think about what muscles you are using. Continue starting and stopping until your flow is finished. Stay on the toilet and continue to contract and release these muscles. The next step is to try to isolate these muscles when you are not urinating. The great thing about pelvic floor exercises is that they can be done anywhere, and no one will notice.

URINARY TRACT INFECTIONS

Most women will experience a UTI (urinary tract infection) sometime during their lifetime. But for some women (one in five) this painful infection can become recurrent, and a vicious cycle of reinfection occurs. Infections are more common with pregnancy, menopause, diabetes, MS and other urinary issues such as using a catheter or having kidney stones. Unfortunately, many cases are triggered by sexual activity.

Signs and symptoms of urinary tract infections include:
- Pain, stinging or a burning sensation with urination (I've heard it explained as feeling like peeing out razor blades).
- A feeling of urgency and frequency with urination (and not much urine coming out).
- Some women experience fatigue and fever, including other general signs of infections.
- Urine might look different; it could be cloudy, dirty, dark and strange smelling. If you have blood in it, head straight to see your GP.
- Pain in your lower abdomen or lower back.
- Some women have minimal symptoms and simply discover an infection with routine testing.

Prevention is definitely better than cure. Here are a few ideas to help you prevent an infection in the first place:

- Wipe front to back! Hopefully, your parents taught you this as a child, but just in case, after every trip to the toilet, you should wipe from your front to your back. This prevents bacteria getting to your urethra.
- If possible, consider showering (cleaning your genitals) before and after sex.
- Make sure you are well lubricated for sex (dryness downstairs is one of the reasons UTI risk can increase with menopause).
- Urinate after sex. This helps flush bacteria out and away from your urethra.
- Are you using contraception? Certain oral contraceptive pills can make you more susceptible to infections. So can a poorly-fitted diaphragm.
- Wear cotton underwear and consider wearing nothing underneath when at home. It's good to let the air circulate down there. If you have a private yard or balcony or if you like nudist beaches, fresh air and sunshine are even better. My old university lecturer swore by sunshine therapy as a treatment for a UTI or even candida.
- Avoid wearing stockings/tights or living in active wear (they block air flow!).
- Avoid very tight clothes such as jeans.
- Empty your bladder frequently and completely.
- Stay well hydrated.
- Have showers instead of baths and look at your soap or body wash. It's best to use a natural product like goat's milk soap without fragrances or chemicals.
- Check that all your female hygiene products (if you still use them) are organic. Cotton is one of the most heavily sprayed crops. You don't want to be putting pesticides directly on your genitals. If you are using incontinence products consider buying organic machine washable pads,

e.g., organic continence pads,[23] disposable organic pads,[24] or reusable underwear.[25]

Diet for prevention and treatment:

- Processed carbohydrates (bread, pasta, cereal, cakes) and sugars feed infection, so avoid like the plague.
- Protein (meat, eggs, tofu, nuts, seeds, fish, chicken) builds immune cells and fights infections, so eat a protein source in every meal.
- Good fats (avocado, eggs, coconut, olive, seafood) helps reduce inflammation and pain.
- Cranberry juice but only the sugar-free variety found in a health food store, not in a supermarket. This prevents bacteria from sticking to the bladder wall. Bacteria need somewhere to attach, to be able to divide and replicate. Therefore, the juice flushes it out and the infection is over. Cranberry contains the active ingredients proanthocyanidins and D-mannose. D-mannose is also found in blueberries, apples, peaches and oranges. Other foods that contain proanthacyanidins include bilberries, strawberries and grapes.
- Probiotic-containing foods such as fermented food help prevent infections by increasing the good bacteria available.
- Water! This may seem like a catch-22, as the last thing you want to do is urinate again due to the burning sensation. However, you need to drink heaps of water to flush out the infection.
- Eat lots of immune boosting foods such as garlic.
- Increase alkaline foods, e.g., fruits, salads and vegetables. The more acidic your body is, the more prone to infection it is.

Additional supplements to consider for an infection:

- High-dose cranberry tablets or straight D-mannose product.
- High-dose immune enhancing probiotics.

---

23. HestaOrganic, 2017. https://www.hestaorganic.com/incontinence-pads
24. Australian Organic Products, 2019. https://australianorganicproducts.com.au/ products/natracare-dry-light-incontinence-pads
25. Modibodi, 2019. https://www.modibodi.co.uk/incontinence-underwear

- Herbal medicine combination that includes a combination of urinary tonics, antiseptics, anti-inflammatories and diuretics (such as alfalfa, bearberry, celery seeds, dandelion, chamomile, chickweed, cornsilk, couch grass, echinacea, goldenrod, horse-chestnut, juniper, marshmallow, parsley, slippery elm, thyme, yarrow).
- Magnesium, if you are experiencing lots of cramping pain.
- Antioxidants and immune enhancers like zinc and vitamin C.

HEADACHES AND MIGRAINES

Fluctuating hormone levels can contribute towards increased headaches and migraines around perimenopause and menopause. If you suffered from hormonal headaches during your fertile years you are at a higher risk of head pain now. But in postmenopause, hormonal headaches may go away altogether as the hormones are lower in general and not fluctuating.

What you probably know is that headaches and migraines are multi-factorial. Yours may be hormone-related but other factors may also contribute to the degree and frequency. It's worth keeping a headache diary and looking at the frequency and timing to help determine what other factors play a role in your discomfort.

Before you blame hormones for your headaches or migraines, you need to rule out some of the other common causes, such as:

- **Dehydration.** This is a common cause of headaches. It's easy to be busy and forget to drink enough water. You need to drink at least 2 litres of water daily, more with exercise.
- **Lack of sleep.** Sleep deprivation can cause many issues and headaches is amongst them. You need 8 hours of uninterrupted sleep. It's not just getting enough sleep that matters, it's also the quality. I know for myself I sometimes get headaches if my sleep was disturbed during the night.

- **Sinus issues.** Sinus congestion and infections are big contributors to headaches. If this is you, it's best to work on improving your sinus health. Start with looking at your diet. Are you eating lots of mucus-forming foods such as dairy? Have you tried a neti pot (a traditional Ayurveda sinus rinsing technique)? Do you need extra probiotics? Those good friendly bacteria live in all mucous membranes and help reduce and fight infection. Are you being exposed to mould in your home, workplace or car? Then consider whether you need herbal help. There are so many herbs that help improve the health of your sinuses. Eyebright is one of my favourites.
- **Eye issues.** When was your last eye test? It may be time for glasses or even different lenses. Some people find sunlight exposure causes headaches. Have you been wearing sunglasses or not? For others, it can be that they have been working too hard and focusing on one point, such as a computer screen for too long. Think of this as an extreme workout for your eyes. You would stretch your leg muscles out after a run, so are you stretching out your eye muscles after a day of work? To do this, sit down and look up as far up as you can and hold your eyes there for the count of 20. Next, move your line of vision to 45 degrees to the right, then hold and count. Next move to as far right as you can, hold and count. Can you feel that stretch? Carry on another 45 degrees, downwards, hold and count. Then look down, hold and stretch. Now repeat everything on the left. If your job involves a lot of looking at screens, you should try to repeat this roughly three times a day.

eye stretching

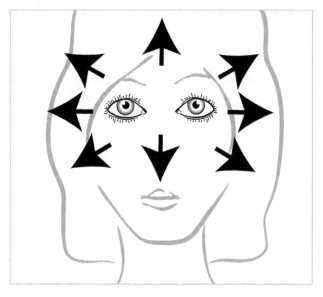

- **Ear issues.** For example, constant ringing from tinnitus would surely give you a headache.
- **Infections/fever.** Infections of any kind can cause headaches. Some cause one off headaches together with other signs of a temporary infection, while others cause more chronic headaches such as long-term residents like herpes simplex 1 and epstein barr virus. If your headache is a one off, temperature is extreme and you have a stiff neck, it might be best to head to hospital and rule out meningitis.
- **Teeth or jaw issues.** These may include clenching or grinding teeth, misaligned bite, impacted wisdom teeth or dental abscesses. Did you know you swallow over 2000 times a day, every day! Therefore, it's not surprising when people with misaligned bites get regular headaches—those

poor overworked muscles are being pulled in unnatural ways too many times a day. If you think this could be you, a dentist or chiropractor may be able to help you further.

- **Neck/shoulder tension.** The good old tension headache. Often described as a band-like sensation around your head that can be mild to moderate in intensity. This is the most common kind. Supplemental magnesium is my go-to for these. Magnesium is a muscle relaxant. Or a massage (I love massages...). Don't forget acupuncture, which almost immediately removes tension headaches. You also need to address several lifestyle factors such as posture or stress levels.
- **Ponytail or other headwear that is too tight.** Yep, this was me as a child. I had such long, thick hair that I had headaches almost every day after school. If you know me, you'll notice to this day, I don't wear my hair up in fear of the dreaded ponytail headache. Luckily removing the hair tie, helmet, cap or other headwear often relieves this type of headache.
- **Food-related headaches.** Food allergies, intolerances and sensitivities can trigger both instant and delayed headaches. Alcohol even falls into this category; some people get an instant headache from the preservatives in red wine, while others can get a delayed headache or a hangover the next day. Caffeine withdrawal is possibly the most common food-related headache. Blood sugar imbalances are also up there as a top contender. Caffeine withdrawal headaches are usually located behind the eyes or frontally located. Blood sugar headaches (can be high or low sugar) are usually located at the base of your skull.
- **Environmental factors.** Radiation and 'dirty energy' can certainly cause headaches. Think about where you are when you get headaches. Are you mostly at home, at work or another location? Consider getting a certified building biologist to come and take a reading of that location and

see if this is a potential problem for you. While they are there, get them to look for mould. Not all mould can be seen or smelt. It's more likely to show up in an area that has previously had water damage.

- **Brain pathology.** Depending on your pattern and severity of pain, your doctor may choose to send you for a brain MRI to rule out pathological causes.

In general, most headaches or migraines improve with these supplements:

- Magnesium (muscle relaxant)
- B2 (riboflavin)
- CoQ10 (ubiquinone or ubiquinol).

Many women find they have a combination of causes for their headaches or migraines. If you are still suffering once you have addressed the above causes, the most likely reason is hormonal imbalances. This imbalance is mostly to do with fluctuating estrogen levels. Therefore, perimenopause with its associated change in hormonal levels can trigger increased issues. Post menopause on the other hand, is generally a pain-free time.

Here are a few supplements to help reduce hormonal headaches or migraines. These suggestions help regulate estrogen levels and have been found to help reduce hormonal headaches and migraines.

- NAC (N Acetyl Cysteine)
- Calcium d glucarate
- Glucoraphanin (broccoli sprouts)
- Turmeric.

WEIGHT

Weight gain is one of the most common complaints of perimenopause, but it doesn't need to be. Just like the rest of your menopausal symptoms, your weight gain—or in some women, the weight redistribution that is primarily around your abdomen—has more to do with ageing, diet, lifestyle, environment and genetics, and less to do with hormonal changes. Consider the following factors as influencing your weight.

Dehydration. It is a well-known fact that the body can confuse the sensation of thirst for hunger, encouraging you to eat more than you need to. Whenever you are hungry, make sure to drink a glass of water first and see if you are still hungry afterwards. Dehydration also slows down your metabolism. Did you know that drinking two glasses of water alone can increase your metabolism by 30%? Finally, dehydration increases the burden on the kidneys. This can affect how the liver functions, as they are both elimination channels. We have already discussed how we need the liver to be functioning at its best. Being well hydrated helps the liver flush any extra toxins from the body.

Lack of sleep impacts negatively on your fat loss attempts as it increases ghrelin and reduces leptin. Let me explain what this means. Ghrelin stimulates appetite, while leptin works in reverse to tell the body to stop eating, by increasing the sensation of fullness. Therefore not only are you tired, but you are also hungrier and eat more as you don't feel full. Sleep deprivation also increases our stress hormone, cortisol, which can increase cravings for sugary foods. Prolonged sleep deprivation (longer than four days), has been found to increase insulin resistance—setting you up for obesity and diabetes, making weight loss even harder. If getting or staying asleep is an issue for you, you may like to check out the section on sleep found in the 'Exercise and other lifestyle factors' chapter.

Cortisol is the stress hormone that makes fat loss difficult. Cortisol's job is to mobilise glycogen stores (short-term energy stores) and increase blood sugar levels. You can only utilise fat stores if there isn't enough energy available. Therefore, in times of stress, you shut down fat loss attempts and start plateauing. Unfortunately for most people, they don't just stop losing fat, they can actually start gaining it! This is because when your blood sugar levels are high, this is followed by a blood sugar low—and lows create a vicious cycle of cravings, especially for sugary type food.

Turning the table on your weight issues begins with determining where you are. Jump on the scales and grab a tape measure. (If you have the interactive version, you can download this page).

measurement chart

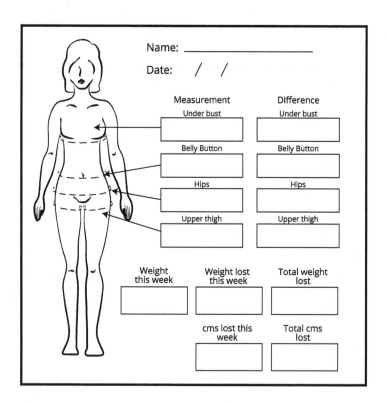

Write a diet diary. It may surprise you just how much you eat and the amount of junk food that sneaks in. Meal planners can also be beneficial. If you plan to eat well, you are halfway there. I personally use a meal planner, so I know what shopping I need to buy, and it also helps to minimise waste. There is a diet diary template and sample seven-day meal planner available on the interactive version.

Remember a flat stomach is made in the kitchen and not in the gym. Food regulates 80% of your weight, and the remaining 20% is exercise. You can't out run a poor diet.

Being overweight increases your need for all antioxidants. Antioxidants include but are not limited to vitamins A, C, E and minerals zinc and selenium. Obesity is also linked to vitamin D deficiency. The larger you are, the more vitamin D you need.

Checklist for finding your ideal size:

1. **Set a realistic target and time frame.** For example, 1 kilogram in a fortnight. If you have lots of weight to lose, chunk it down into achievable amounts and celebrate your accomplishments. Reward yourself with non-food prizes, such as buying yourself a new dress when you drop a size
2. **Plan to eat well.** Go back and read the 'Ultimate Checklist for INVINCIBLE Eating' section. Add to this a diet diary or meal planner to track what you actually eat.
3. **Motivate yourself for success.** Hang an old favourite item of clothing that no longer fits you and try it on once a week. Watch it get closer and closer to fitting. Find old pictures of yourself that you both love and hate the way you look and put them on the fridge. This might help you choose to feed the healthier version of yourself and not the unhealthy version of you.
4. **Recruit a friend or two.** Friends can support you on your weight loss journey. Share your challenges, keep everyone accountable and celebrate your wins together. If your friends are more likely to sabotage your success than encourage you,

it's time to look for support elsewhere. You may benefit from the support of a practitioner, or your local area may have suitable group activities such as walking groups where you can meet new people who value health.

5. **Open up your elimination pathways.** Old body fat doesn't just evaporate, it needs to be removed from your body. You need to be well hydrated. Expect increased urination and bowel movements. If you are constipated go back and read the section on 'Digestive issues'. Constipation will slow down your results and needs to be addressed.

6. **Increase lymphatic movement.** Your lymphatic system works like a sewer; it moves around and removes waste products. Increasing the movement of lymphatic fluid cleanses the body and increases its ability to drop weight. Try dry skin brushing, massage and movement. Why not head to the day spa? This can be a good reward for hitting your first target and help accelerate the arrival of your next weight goal.

7. **Sleep.** Make sure you are getting enough sleep.

8. **Stress less.** Manage your stress levels.

9. **Exercise.** This is essential but start where you are at. Don't run your first marathon if you haven't run in years. Start somewhere and build on that over time.

10. **Supplemental help.** Consider whether the following supplements could be of benefit to you in reaching your goal. This is number ten for a reason; it should be the last thing you consider after you have tweaked your diet and exercise regime.

    - Beneficial fats can help burn bad fats, e.g., MCT oil.
    - Liver support, such as milk thistle and dandelion.
    - Fat transporter, such as choline, inositol or carnitine.
    - Blood sugar regulator/craving support, such as chromium.
    - Digestive support such as probiotics, enzymes and apple cider vinegar capsules.

Supplemental 'don't includes' are fat absorbing supplements like chitosan, as it also absorbs all of your good fat-soluble nutrients at the same time. Avoid products with lots of stimulants in them, like caffeine. It's OK to use natural caffeine such as that found in green tea, but the amount found in weight loss supplements is over the top.

BLOOD GLUCOSE

With the reduction of estrogen, also comes an increased risk of Type 2 diabetes. Estrogen supports the pathways that regulate insulin and blood glucose. Nothing is more important than a whole food diet as described in the 'Nutritious foods' section. Regular exercise and adequate sleep are also essential.

Did you know that it's possible to get diabetes even with a decent diet? Excessive stress can also contribute to this diagnosis. So, the importance of lifestyle factors to reduce your stress response are vital components needed to win the battle against sugar. When you are stressed, your body produces additional cortisol. This hormone liberates stored sugar into active blood sugar to provide you with energy to run away from danger. Have you ever been that stressed that you feel shaky? This is the stress response telling you to run and escape the stressor. If you don't burn this additional sugar, insulin is produced to store it away again for another day. If this keeps happening, it can lead to insulin resistance or prediabetes.

Blood sugar imbalances produce similar symptoms as the menopausal transition. If you are experiencing any or all of these symptoms you need to rule out blood sugar irregularities before putting all the blame on your hormones:
- hot flushes
- fatigue
- brain fog
- weight gain

- issues getting to sleep
- issues staying asleep
- bad moods (irritable, aggressive, snappy)
- recurrent headaches
- digestive issues
- frequent infections
- feeling short of breath
- skin outbreaks
- inflammation and pain
- feeling dizzy
- trembling hands
- hair loss.

These are the tests I recommend to help you assess how balanced your blood sugar levels are. Please note these must be tested in a FASTING state.

- Glucose – active blood sugar level
- Insulin – this hormone is released when carbohydrates are ingested or when call upon by your cortisol – your stress hormones. Insulin signals for the storage of sugars and the stockpiling of fats.
- HbA1c – Glycated hemoglobin. Hemoglobin is a protein found in red blood cells. When glucose builds up in your blood it binds to hemoglobin. This test measures how much glucose is bound. As red blood cells live for about 3 months, this test shows the average level of glucose in your blood over the past 3 months.

An additional test to have is a hair tissue mineral analysis (HTMA) to check for toxic metals. Diabetics have an increased tendency to absorb and store metals. Alternatively, you can check your blood for iron overload or elevated copper. These two imbalances are common with both menopause and diabetes, and if you have both your risk is even higher.

If you have already developed diabetes, it's important to be aware that the menopausal transition will play havoc on your blood sugar readings. Some women will require additional medications or increased doses of their existing medication to stabilise their readings at this time.

Did you realise Type 2 diabetes is reversible? It's a lifestyle disease that if left unchecked will gradually get worse, requiring more and more drugs. Or if you prefer, you can turn this disease around with lots of work and effort. A lifestyle disease can be corrected by generally doing the opposite to what gave you the disease in the first place. So, replacing inactivity with regular exercise, replacing sleepless nights with adequate rest or replacing processed foods with organic meals high in protein, good fats and vegetables. It's your life, so it's your choice.

Supplements to consider:
- Chromium – reduces cravings and enhances the action of insulin
- Inositol – reduces blood glucose
- Vitamin D – deficiency is linked to metabolic syndrome, it also helps prevent diabetes
- Resveratrol – reduces the accelerated ageing response from high blood glucose
- Alpha-lipoic acid – this antioxidant protects against free radical damage and is especially important if you are diabetic. It can prevent and treat peripheral neuropathy. I've seen it work wonders with diabetic-related foot issues.
- Magnesium – helps reduce cravings, helps balance blood sugar levels and diabetes have a higher need for magnesium.

Herbs to consider:
- Gymnema – this is an Indian herb also called "the sugar destroyer".
- Cinnamon – increases insulin sensitivity and lowers blood sugar levels.

THYROID

Your thyroid gland regulates the body's metabolic rate as well as cardiovascular risk, digestive function, muscle control, brain development, mood, bone turnover and longevity. What an important organ!

Unfortunately, your thyroid is more likely to play up as you age. With one in 12 women struggling in perimenopause and one in six women with thyroid issues post menopause. That's huge! Hypothyroidism (underactive thyroid) is by far the most common thyroid issue. However, hyperthyroidism, nodular thyroid disease and thyroid cancer are also at an increased risk as you age. As hypothyroidism is the most common, it's what I'll focus on in this section. Signs and symptoms of an underactive thyroid are very similar to menopause and as a result, often go undiagnosed.

Signs and symptoms
- Fatigue
- Brain fog
- Weight gain
- Hair loss
- Brittle nails
- Constipation
- Dry skin
- Irritable moods/mood swings/depression
- Low libido.

Due to the similarities and the increased frequency of thyroid issues, it is very important to test your thyroid function thoroughly. Determine if your symptoms are menopause or thyroid related, as you won't get a long-term result until you determine the underlying cause of your problem and work specifically on that.

Testing

The tests I recommend include:

- TSH: thyroid stimulating hormone (encourages the conversion of T4 to T3)
- Free T4
- Free T3
- Reverse T3
- Thyroid antibodies, e.g., thyroid peroxidase antibodies (TPO), thyroglobulin antibodies (TGAb), thyroid receptor antibodies (TRAb)
- Urinary iodine test
- Vitamin D
- Epstein barr virus, as a lot of auto-immune conditions have links with infections. EBV has an affinity for the thyroid and may be a possible cause for thyroid autoimmunity.
- A thyroid physical exam and or an ultrasound.

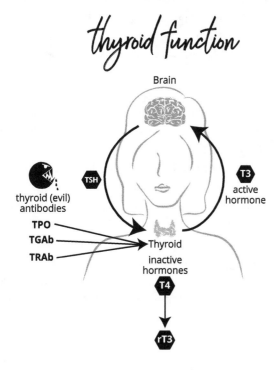

Your brain sends down thyroid stimulating hormone (TSH) to encourage the conversion of T4 (inactive thyroid hormone) into T3 (active thyroid hormone). T3 then sends a feedback message to the brain to say, 'Thanks we have enough, you need to reduce the amount of TSH, all is good here'. However, when T3 levels aren't good, that message doesn't get through and your TSH level gets higher and higher. Under times of stress T4 is sent down different pathways and produces rT3 (also inactive) instead of T3. This also prevents the feedback message and TSH can rise. Thyroid antibodies should be investigated as well. These can start to elevate a decade before the thyroid is damaged—enough to stop converting T4 to T3 and for blood tests to indicate an issue by looking at abnormal TSH levels. It's like trying to complete a jigsaw puzzle without all the pieces. It's worth paying for private testing so you can see the entire picture.

Essential nutrients for optimal thyroid function include:
- Iodine is a key building block of T3 and T4. The numbers 3 and 4 correspond to the numbers of iodine molecules on the thyroid hormone. Don't take in the presence of thyroid antibodies unless under the care of a healthcare practitioner.
- Zinc is needed for the formation of thyroid hormones.
- Selenium is needed for the conversion of T4 (inactive thyroid hormone) to T3 (active).
- Tyrosine along with iodine is a key building block to form thyroid hormones.
- Magnesium helps build T4, convert T4 to T3 and prevent goiter alongside iodine.
- Vitamin D is a key component of T reg cells, which regulate the thyroid. It can also reduce elevated TSH.
- Vitamin A can help reduce the formation of a goiter, reduce thyroid antibodies and improve thyroid function in women with hypothyroidism.

- Probiotics (yes there is also a Gut-Thyroid connection). The best strains include saccharomyces boulardii and lactobacillus or bifidum species.
- B12 is often reduced in patients with hypothyroidism.
- Manganese helps transport T4 in the cells (T4 is converted to T3 inside the cells).

It is essential to clean up your diet if you have a thyroid condition. Some foods known as goitrogens further reduce the functioning of your thyroid. These include raw cruciferous vegetables, e.g., bok choy, broccoli, cauliflower, kale, cabbage and spinach. These can be deactivated by cooking. Soy products such as tofu and tempeh also contain goitrogenic compounds and should be avoided.

It's also a good time to remind you that some of the dietary recommendations discussed in the 'Nutritious food' section are even more important if your thyroid isn't optimally functioning. These include avoiding gluten, dairy, soy and sugar.

SKIN

Although ageing skin is not a disease or a medical condition that requires treatment, it is something that worries many women and can impact on their self-esteem and mental health. There are skin conditions such as rosacea and acne that are more commonly triggered during this time and may require additional help.

AGEING SKIN

Hormonal changes during menopause also affect your skin. With the reduction of estrogen happening faster than testosterone, adult acne can occur. This is because testosterone stimulates sebaceous glands to produce a thicker sebum that can cause oily facial skin and acne. Relative testosterone dominance (higher ratio but not necessarily high reading) is also the cause of those unwanted new chin hairs.

The reduction of estrogen also causes fat redistribution. Increased fat deposits around your abdomen, hips and thighs and away from other areas like your face, neck and breasts. The reduction of these supportive fat deposits in these areas causes sagging skin, wrinkles and line development.

Estrogen reduction is also responsible for the reduction of collagen levels and elastin levels. Collagen and elastin are also less able to repair themselves without the stimulation of estrogen. Collagen provides your skin with structure, while elastin allows your skin to stretch and move. The reduction of these two proteins encourages the sagging and ageing of your skin.

Glycosaminoglycans are essential for skin hydration as they increase water retention in the skin. As estrogen levels reduce so do these and your skin starts to become drier in general, as it cannot maintain hydration in the skin.

The epidermal layer of skin starts to thin. This is due to the reduction of blood capillaries that provide oxygen and other nutrients to the skin. The growth and maintenance of the blood capillaries are linked with estrogen levels. Therefore, your skin becomes thinner and drier and more prone to damage. This damage takes longer to heal as your skin isn't receiving as many nutrients to encourage healing. This same process is occuring in your vagina and urinary tract, which is why you may also experience vaginal dryness and be more at risk of urinary tract infections.

Have you started noticing tiny white dots on your arms or legs? Melanocytes are the cells that produce the pigment melanin. These are the cells that give your skin the tanned look after spending time in the sun. Melanocytes are regulated by estrogen. Too little and you may start noticing a few white dots here and there on areas that have previously been exposed to the sunlight. Too much and you start developing skin pigmentation. Have you ever noticed the majority of pigmentation occurs on your face and hands, the two areas that have been exposed to sunlight the most over your life?

Healthy skin ageing starts with the right diet and lifestyle factors as discussed before, but I would like to highlight the importance of a few factors such as drinking enough water and eating enough protein. Protein is essential as its the starting block for building new collagen. You need an abundance of antioxidant rich fruit and vegetables as these protect your skin from free radical damage. Key antioxidants include:

- Vitamin C is needed in the production of collagen.
- Vitamin D is critical for new skin development and repair.
- Vitamin E inhibits free radical damage.
- Zinc is another essential building block for new skin development and repair.

You should also consume a lot of beneficial oils such as seafood, avocado and eggs; good oils help to lubricate your skin from the inside out. If you are considering supplements, fish oils are good, but sea buckthorn is better. Sea buckthorn has the added benefit of containing omega 7. Not heard of omega 7? This is particularly beneficial for lubricating dry skin, dry eyes or a dry vagina. This section on skin health wouldn't be complete if I didn't mention probiotics. These good bacteria help improve the function and strength of the skin's natural barrier.

Try your best to avoid inflammatory foods such as those you are sensitive or allergic to, and processed foods and sugars. These cause free-radical damage to your skin and are linked with dark circles under your eyes, loss of skin tone, puffiness, acne, lines, wrinkles, loss of facial contour, bigger pore sizes and inflamed red and itchy skin. Alcohol can also be detrimental to your skin health. Alcohol causes the small blood vessels in your skin to widen. This may cause the skin to flush and a sensation of warmth to occur. Over time this can lead to broken capillaries on your face. It's also linked to dull or discoloured skin, enlarged pores, skin sag and dry, dehydrated skin. Caffeine can also cause dehydrated skin.

Certain lifestyle factors also impact on skin health; the most notorious is smoking. Smokers have paler skin, more lines and wrinkles than non-smokers. This is partially due to reduced circulation caused by the nicotine. This results in fewer nutrients getting to the skin and a decreased ability of the skin to release its toxic waste products of normal cell metabolism. This makes smokers more prone to skin conditions.

Stress causes the hormone cortisol to be released into the bloodstream. Excess prolonged cortisol causes the skin to thin, wrinkle and makes your blood vessels more visible under the skin. A good night's sleep can help you feel refreshed and look radiant as well. It is needed to avoid eye puffiness. But most importantly it's during sleep that the body, including the skin cells, repair and recover.

Regular exercise shows in your skin too. Research has shown people who maintain their activity levels have thicker skin with increased collagen fibres. Collagen gives the skin its strength and flexibility.

Fun fact

The skin has been called the third kidney because it removes almost as much waste material from the body each day, as the kidneys themselves. Ageing skin can't effectively remove these waste products anymore. Therefore, it's very important to reduce the number of toxins you are exposed to in the first place. Go back and read the section on 'Creating a non-toxic environment' if you need to.

HAIR LOSS

Around 50% of women will experience some form of hair loss during their lifetime, although it's more common later in life. Hair loss is often accompanied with additional stress, anxiety and depression for the women involved. It is also linked with lower self-esteem, a negative body image and self-isolation.

Pattern hair loss in women is the most common and is characterised by excessive hair thinning. This starts in the mid-front hairline and widens. This is different from male pattern hair loss, which starts with a receding hairline.

Potential causes:
- Elevated testosterone (especially DHT form).
- Thyroid dysfunction.
- Parathyroid dysfunction.
- Autoimmune conditions like lupus.
- Diabetes.
- Digestive dysfunction, SIBO, leaky gut and dysbiosis.
- Dietary issues: excessive fasting, protein deficiency, gluten intolerance.
- Stress.
- Genetics.
- Cardiovascular issues e.g., elevated blood pressure, coronary heart disease.
- Chronic inflammation.
- Infections such as syphilis (this looks different as it's more of a patchy hair loss).
- Nutritional deficiencies (common deficiencies include vitamin A, vitamin B complex (Niacin, Biotin, B6, B12), vitamin D, zinc, silica, selenium, iron, iodine, essential fatty acids.)
- Smoking.
- Working long hours under ultraviolet light.
- Toxin exposure, such as heavy metals.

Testing
- Hormones: estradiol, testosterone, dihydrotestosterone (DHT), DHEAs, SHBG, prolactin, progesterone
- Cortisol: saliva test four times during the day is the gold standard, but a morning blood test is a possible starting point.

- Thyroid testing TSH, FT3, FT4, rT3, TPO, TGAb, TRAb, urinary iodine.
- Parathyroid hormone PTH.
- Full blood count.
- Iron/ferritin.
- Zinc.
- Vitamin D.
- ANA (to consider auto-immune component).
- ESR and CRP (inflammatory markers).
- Glucose, insulin, HbA1c.
- Blood pressure.
- Cholesterol.
- HTMA (heavy metal hair test).

Possible treatment options
- Peonia and licorice herbal combination to reduce testosterone levels.
- Saw palmetto to help reduce DHT form of testosterone.
- Cod liver oil is a source of vitamin A, D and essential fatty acids.
- Silica is a building block for new hair.
- NAC (N Acetyl Cysteine) can help balance hormones and reduce hair loss.
- Iron if found to be low.
- Zinc if found to be low.
- Thyroid support if needed.
- Withania to help reduce cortisol levels.
- Inositol for blood sugar support and hormonal balance.
- B complex with high amounts of biotin, niacin, B6, B12 and choline.
- Probiotics (especially L. reuteri strain and Saccharomyces boulardii).

Also consider:

- Counselling, coaching or psychology
- Acupuncture/acupressure
- Scalp massage
- Yoga
- Changing your hair products to low-toxic products and reducing the frequency of washing, brushing and styling.

IMMUNE HEALTH

'An inflammatory state devoid of protective
immune factors characterizes the immune
microenvironment in menopausal women.'[26]

Let's make sure you are the exception and not the rule, in this case.

Yes, as your hormones drop you are more prone to:
• Viral infections and viral reactivation of previous infections.
• Bacterial and other microbial infections.
• Cancer.
• Auto-immune conditions.
• Increased inflammation.

If you have ever doubted the link between your hormones and your immune system think of those poor women that get cyclic thrush infections, cyclic herpes outbreaks or are generally more prone to infections at either ovulation or menstruation—two times of major hormonal change.

Luckily there are many things you can do to protect your immune system and give it a helping hand, no matter what stage of life you are in.

Lifestyle factors to improve immunity include:
• Stressing less.
• Sleeping well.
• Eating well.
• Digesting well and having good bowel movements.
• Breathing well and getting plenty of fresh air.
• Getting adequate sunshine exposure.

26. Ghosh, M., Rodriguez-Garcia, M., and Wira, C.R (2014). The Immune System in Menopause: Pros and Cons of Hormone Therapy. The Journal of Steriod Biochemistry and Molecular Biology 142, 171-175. https://www.ncbi.nlm.nih.gov/pmc/articles/PMC3954964

- Avoiding poor lifestyle choices such as smoking and drinking.
- Improving hygiene factors such as washing your hands.
- Getting the right amount of exercise (underexercise and overexercise are linked with reduced immunity).
- Making sure your body isn't compromised by toxic substances, such as metals or chemicals.
- Avoiding cell damaging radiation and electromagnetic fields.
- Fostering positive, happy thoughts builds a stronger immune system. You know the old saying 'Laughter is the best medicine.'
- Anything that improves lymphatic movement improves your immunity. Consider dry skin brushing, massaging and stretching.
- Acupuncture and chiropractic treatments can also assist your immune system.
- Being your ideal body weight. Obesity increases inflammation and reduces immune function.

Dietary considerations

- Are you eating plenty of fresh fruit and vegetables?
- Are you hydrated? Do you need more water?
- Are you eating adequate protein? Protein is an essential building block for new immune cells.
- Are you avoiding 'bad' processed/heated fats? Are you getting enough good fats?
- Avoid sugar. Sugar feeds the bugs and supports the other team.

FLU BREW

There are many similar varieties. Add what you like, remove what you don't. If I'm at home I load up extra garlic but if I'm making a batch to take to work, I leave the garlic out. Chili may be another ingredient you play with. Always check the potency and dilute as needed. Caution if taking with a high fever.

Ingredients
1L water
5 slices of fresh ginger
1 sliced chili
3 cloves of garlic
Freshly squeezed lemon or lime
1 cinnamon stick
1 tablespoon honey

Directions
1. Place water, ginger, chili, garlic and cinnamon into the saucepan.
2. Bring to the boil, reduce heat and simmer for 10 minutes.
3. Strain and add juice (lemon or lime) and honey to taste.
4. Drink hot.

Any remaining liquid can be added back to ingredients and placed in the fridge and drank later. Warning: the longer you leave the ingredients together the more potent it gets. I highly recommend diluting this remaining batch with water. Another tip is to make a double batch and freeze one, as you never know when you are going to need it next.

SALTWATER GARGLE

Saltwater gargles can help to reduce sore throats and assist in loosening mucus/phlegm lodged in the throat area. Mucus is where bacteria and harmful microbes like to set up shop, so using salt water gargles can help to flush these microbes out of the body to allow for a faster recovery.

Ingredients

1 teaspoon of salt (Celtic Sea salt)
1 cup of warm-hot water

Directions

1. Stir and dissolve 1 teaspoon of salt into the cup of warm-hot water.
2. Pour some of the salt solution into your mouth and while tilting the head back, start to gargle. Continue for about 1 minute and then spit the solution out.
3. Continue to do this until all of the salt solution is gone.
4. Repeat every few hours or as needed.

For more immune boosting home remedies, jump on to the interactive version.

Supplements

- Probiotics: immune protecting, anti-microbial and anti-inflammatory
- Vitamin A: decreases sensitivities to pollutants, acts as an antioxidant, improves mucous membrane integrity, increases lymphocytes (the little pac-men in your body that eat up foreign invaders) and generally increases resistance to infections and cancer.

- Vitamin B5: reduces your body's response to stress, improves energy levels and stimulates antibody production.
- Vitamin C: increases production of natural antibodies especially lymphocytes, acts as a natural antihistamine, is antibacterial, antiviral and an antioxidant.
- Vitamin D: is an immune balancer. It helps prevent infections and reduce auto-immunity.
- Vitamin E: is one of the strongest antioxidants. It works best for prevention and protection.
- Selenium: is needed to make natural antibodies.
- Zinc: is an antioxidant, helps prevent cancer, acts as an antihistamine and acts as a strong immune enhancer by increasing lymphocytes and helper cells. Specifically, antiviral.
- Magnesium: is essential for proper thymus functioning, for the formation of prostaglandins and for controlling histamine levels.
- Calcium: is needed by the T-cells to battle the invading pathogens. It is also needed to enable white blood cells to digest and destroy viruses.
- Manganese: is needed to produce interferon.
- L-lysine: prevents viral replication and speeds up recovery from viral outbreaks.
- Echinacea: probably the best known and most used herb in the Western world. Echinacea is renowned for improving immunity in acute cases and for preventing infections. It is specific for fighting viral or bacterial infection, reducing inflammation, stimulating lymphatic movement and for general healing. What most people don't know is that is also an adaptogen, which means it helps to reduce your stress response.
- Andrographis: an Indian herb that reduces the stress response, reduces inflammation, improves digestion, tones the liver and happens to be one of the strongest immune stimulators known to man. Good for chronic or acute infections.

- Astragalus: not to be used in acute infections. Works well in chronic immune deficiency and also helps reduce the body's response to stress.

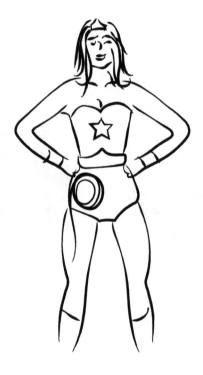

Jennifer is sharing more in her
INTERACTIVE book.

See exclusive, behind-the-scenes
videos, audios and photos.

DOWNLOAD free content and go
From Invisible To Invincible.

deanpublishing.com/invincible

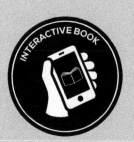

headspace

For the majority of women transitioning into menopause, moods can be a struggle. It is more prevalent with women who have a history of anxiety or depression, but it can affect any woman. Mental health concerns in women tend to peak after puberty and again in perimenopause.

Common feelings include being angry, feeling unable to cope, anxiety, irritability, feeling isolated, depressed, being tearful, feeling flat, lacking joy and being unable to enjoy things that they previously liked. This doesn't sound like fun. Please see below for specific hints and tips to help get you over your hurdle and back to enjoying life. If in doubt, book an appointment to talk to your naturopath, doctor, counsellor or psychologist.

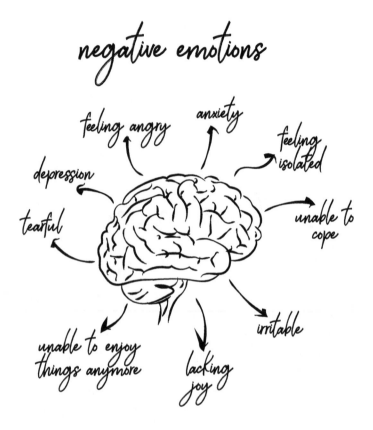

Potential causes of all mood changes

Have you heard of the gut-brain axis? This is the connection between what you eat and how you feel. The biochemical signals that takes place between the gut and the central nervous system.

Remember in the 'Intuition' section I mentioned your digestive system actually makes more neurotransmitters than your brain does? The neurotransmitters involved with mood are serotonin, GABA and noradrenalin, dopamine, glutamate and acetylcholine. Serotonin is coined as your feel-good hormone and 90% of it is produced in your digestive system. Therefore, digestive issues can reduce the amount of serotonin available from the gut and change your mood.

There is also a brain-gut axis where your thoughts affect how your digestion functions. Most of us have at some point experienced butterflies before an important event or even had diarrhoea. This is a two-way street. Consider the state of your diet. Have you implemented all the diet changes mentioned above? Have you cut out sugar, gluten and dairy? Are you eating enough protein and beneficial fats? Do you have additional food sensitivities outside of the common ones that need identifying and eliminating? On top of diet, I would add in a mood specific probiotic, alternatively called psychobiotics. These are a family of probiotics that enhance the gut-brain axis and specifically improve mood.

Mood changes can be thought of as inflammation in your brain. The blood test CRP (c-reactive protein) is a marker of systemic inflammation which may be handy, whereas an Organic Acids Tests (OAT) specifically measures quinolinate levels.

Quinolinate is a direct marker of brain inflammation and is a known cause of mood disorders, fatigue, sleep disturbance, withdrawal, no libido, appetite changes, cognitive issues and the inability to experience joy. If your levels are high, your poor brain is on fire! Women with mood disorders and elevated inflammatory markers do not respond to traditional antidepressant medication. Instead, they need anti-inflammatory assistance—or a call to the fire department. Throw anti-inflammatory oils like fish oil over it immediately, and then find some saffron and turmeric. The kitchen herbs taste nice, but in the case of severe mood disorders I would bypass these and start a supplement version straight away. These herbs both put out the fire and protect the brain from the flames.

Estrogen modulates production of serotonin and dopamine. Therefore, a decrease in estrogen can cause your moods to come crashing down. As previously discussed, serotonin also has a role to play in raising estrogen levels and this is why antidepressants are sometimes prescribed in menopause.

Progesterone, or more so, lack of progesterone, may also be a causative factor here. The act of ovulation produces progesterone and when your ovaries stop regularly ovulating each month, this hormone drops. Progesterone is converted to allopregnanolone in the brain, which is known for its calming, anti-anxiety and memory-enhancing effects. Hence, this might be when your first round of symptoms occur. The most common symptom being that you are now potentially more prone to anxiety, unable to sleep as well as you used to and possibly have night sweats. Although everyone is different, this is the most common pattern I see in practice.

ANXIETY

Personally, this is something I first experienced in early perimenopause. Having not suffered from anxiety before, it came as a surprise. But it wasn't 100% out-of-the-blue; in my case, it was a response to a stressful time in my life. Things that wouldn't have worried me before, became a big issue and everything escalated from there. You might find your anxiety also has triggers, or you might not.

Women with anxiety can experience palpitations, dry mouth, digestive issues, muscle tension, headache, insomnia, flushes and crawling skin, whether they are going through menopause or not. A few sleepless nights, and little problems become big problems, which can also trigger anxiety, regardless of your hormonal status.

Here are a few tips of things to do when experiencing anxiety

- Exercise. Exercise helps to settle the mind. Instinctively our body knows this, and some women will naturally start to pace or go for a longer walk. Exercising during a moment of anxiety is like a band-aid—it can help at the moment, but regular exercise will help prevent or reduce your anxiety spells.

- Breathe. You've got this. Go back to the section on 'Breathe' and make sure you implement as much as possible.
- Switch off the TV and stop listening to or reading the news. Being bombarded with bad news all the time is setting the scene for anxiety.
- Be in nature. Out in the sunshine. Sunlight exposure is so beneficial for healthy happy moods. Watch the sunrise, sunset, watch the stars, watch the clouds float by, watch a storm, stop and smell the flowers, do some gardening, go bird watching, earth yourself – take off your shoes and walk barefoot in nature. Go Forest bathing (Shrinrin-yoku), a Japanese form of just taking in the forest atmosphere.
- Get wet. Floating is my kind of meditation; other women find swimming their way of calming and clearing their mind. You might love a long soak in the bath.
- If you prefer to stay dry, just watching the waves crash to shore can be therapeutic. Some women find sailing therapeutic, or even just catching a ferry relaxing. Padding is another suggestion, whether it be on a stand-up paddleboarding or kayaking is another favourite of mine.
- Music. Can you play an instrument? Taking time out to play can be fun and relaxing. If you can't play an instrument you can still enjoy music, sing like no one is listening, dance like no one is watching and let the rhythm move you.
- Art. Get your easel out and draw something. If you aren't artistic consider visiting a gallery and admiring other people's art. Make something e.g., knit, sew, crochet, quilt, do flower decoration. Join a class and learn how to create something new.
- Pet therapy. I'm a dog lover but spending time with any kind of pet helps to calm your nerves.
- Reading, it doesn't matter the genre. I love inspiring non-fiction type books, but anything you don't want to put down counts as a stress management tool.
- Play games; board games, card games, etc. I personally love backgammon.

- Visualisations or guided imagery meditations are very effective tools.
- Affirmations when said regularly can get you in a better state of mind. "I am enough. I am worthy. I am loveable. I am excited about today."
- Journaling, which can be written or drawn. Taking the time to document what is going on in your life and how you are feeling.
- Probably one of the most valuable activities is gratitude. Regularly take the time to think about and thank about all the wonderful things that are happening for you. It's not possible to be anxious and grateful at the same time!

Nutritionally, you may need more magnesium. Magnesium is a muscle relaxant. It can help you calm down and is also good for insomnia, headaches and muscle aches. Other nutrients to consider include B complex and vitamin C.

Here are a few herbs to consider for anxiety:
- Kava: reduces anxiety, aids sleep, reduces stress and is a muscle relaxant.
- Lavender: helps improve mood and sleep. It can also reduce headaches.
- Motherwort: when anxiety is accompanied with palpitations or angina.
- Passionflower: helps with anxiety, restlessness, headaches and nerve pain.
- Lemon balm: reduces anxiety and anxiety related digestive issues.
- St John's Wort: anxiety, depression, nerve pain, insomnia, antiviral. Specific herb for menopausal moods but interacts with prescription medicine so speak to your health care provider before trialling this. Can also cause photosensitivity.

- Black Cohosh: can reduce anxiety and depression when related to hormonal change. Another specific herb for menopausal moods.
- Valerian: reduces anxiety and anxiety related sleep disturbances.
- Zizyphus: my favourite herb for anxiety. It can also reduce menopausal symptoms such as night sweats.

DEPRESSION

Considerations for lifting you out of your depression and creating more joy:

- Sleep. Not having a good night's sleep for days, weeks or months can feel like depression. Dragging yourself around and having a generally lower interest in life. If this is you, you don't need anti-depressants, you need a good night's sleep.
- Orgasm. Dr Christiane Northrup, relates depression in menopause with a lack of orgasms. She often sends women away with a script for at least three orgasms a week. She doesn't mind if it's with your partner or by yourself. If you are still depressed after this, the real scripts come out. I dare you to try it! What do you have to lose?
- Exercise is another lifestyle factor that can dramatically transform your moods.
- Smokers are more prone to depression than non-smokers.
- Empty nests can cause loneliness and looking after ageing parents can be difficult. Many relationships break down during this time. This stage of life offers many challenges. Don't be afraid to reach out for help.

Tried and tested supplementation for depression include magnesium, fish oil, Vitamin D and a B complex.

These herbs may also be of benefit:

- Ginseng family can be useful if mood changes are accompanied with physical exhaustion.
- Lavender, if your depression is accompanied with insomnia and headaches.
- Oats, if your depression is accompanied with exhaustion.
- Rosemary, for depression with mental impairment and headache.
- Saffron improves mood by reducing inflammation (remember quinolinate?). It may also be an aphrodisiac and is great in combination with turmeric.
- Skullcap, for depression with insomnia, headache and nerve pain.
- St John's Wort is a specific herb for depression in menopause (see caution in 'Anxiety' section).
- Turmeric, specific for pain related depression. Improves mood by reducing inflammation.
- Withania is the ultimate chill herb, but more so for stress and exhaustion than depression.

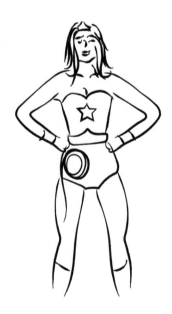

begin your transformation today

Congratulations on reading this far, it's almost the end. I just wanted to make sure you know where to start and how to start taking action so that you too can become INVINCIBLE!

Have you taken the quiz? Here is the link again just in case.

https://www.menopausenaturalsolutions.com/menopause-symptom-tracker-quiz

Once you start making changes, go back and re-do the quiz.

Remember, healing is not a linear process. It may have its ups and downs or may even change course. Healing is often referred to as being like an onion; one layer improves and then a new layer shows up. Don't be put off by this. Take the common cold as an example. It may start as a sore throat, move into a fever, then into a cough or sinus issue. Movement is a good sign of progression towards healing.

If you want to start transforming, start with the 10 INVINCIBLE steps. If you have any symptoms remaining, then move to the specific areas.

Remember that this book is the starting point. The interactive version of the book expands on this content and includes:

- Meal planner and recipes.
- Additional information about the investigations and reference ranges.
- Additional information about environmental health
- Extra breathing exercises and meditations.

And more.

LET'S STAY CONNECTED

If you'd like to reach out further, please check out my website: menopausenaturalsolutions.com

On the website, you can:
- Complete the quiz
- Sign up for my newsletter
- Join an in-person health retreat and have a wonderful healing holiday
- Join our online retreat and enjoy the benefits of this community from the comfort of your own home.

For the ultimate Menopause Makeover, start working one-on-one with my naturopaths. This is the express option for the ultimate health transformation.

My Facebook page
facebook.com/menopausenaturalsolutions

My Podcast

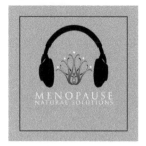

I want to wish you all the best in your journey to true health and happiness.

I hope our paths cross again, until then.

Much love,

Jen

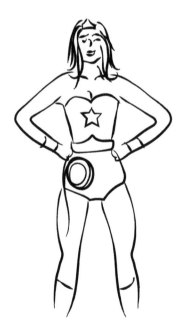

acknowledgements

I would like to start by thanking all of my patients; past, present and future. Without you, I wouldn't be the practitioner that I am. It doesn't matter how many years you spend in university, without people willing to put their trust in you, you can't grow and evolve as a professional; and this is what I think sets me apart from many of my fellow naturopaths — the sheer numbers of patients I've consulted with. My patients have taught me more about naturopathy and life than I could have ever learnt in university. Thank you!

To the pioneers of Functional Medicine, thanks for allowing me to stand on your shoulders. There is one doctor who has inspired me more than anyone else and although I have never met Dr Christiane Northrup I want to acknowledge her work as a major source of inspiration for me.

I wouldn't still be practising today if I didn't have the opportunities I had as a new graduate. I'm extremely grateful for the team at Chiva Som International Health Resort – for giving me a go. Under the guidance of Jeff Nieuwenhuizen and the support of the entire team special thanks to Sue Davis,

Karen Ansell, Eliza Blackwood, Kelli Chinn, Nun Nuntawadee, and Orranat Thanamteun.

To my team at Parramatta Naturopathic Clinic, thank you for believing in me and my vision for the clinic. Thanks to John Miller Crispe for taking the baton from me and continuing to grow my dream after I've left. Special thanks go to Amanda Morley, Nicola Kelly, Thie Sakae, Carolyn Frasche, Helen Laws, Tiffany Baxter, and Soo Liang Ooi for being a part of my dream team.

To Anne-Marijke Gerretsen, it has been an absolute joy watching you evolve, from a patient, to a student and then to a practitioner. I'm extremely thankful for the hundreds of hours you spent helping me with research for this book. I would still be in the research stage now if you hadn't of helped me out.

To the Natural Fertility Breakthrough Crew. A big thank you to Alison Cassar, you were so generous with sharing your knowledge. I also want to thank Gabriela Rosa, Nicola Andrews, Georgia Hartman, Jo Lia, Jo Wilson and Ann Bridges. The combined knowledge of this clinic is mind-blowing.

There wouldn't be a chapter in this book on "Contribution" if it wasn't for Dale Beaumont from Business Blueprint. Not only did Dale teach me how to go from a passionate practitioner to a business owner but he also instilled the value of giving back. His involvement with Hands Across the Water is inspiring. Thank you for letting me accompany you on not only 1 but 2 journeys across Thailand. And my fellow cyclists (now lifetime friends), although our bottoms were very sore from the gruelling +500km rides, and the triple whammy of hills, heat and humidity, our hearts were filled with an indescribable joy that can only come from giving.

I have so much gratitude for my Blueprint coach Cameron Quinn who encouraged me to create my own community and planted the first seed for the Online Retreat. I am also extremely grateful to my accountability buddy, the very talented Darryl Lovegrove.

Another extremely talented friend is Jannet Serhan from printandproper (www.printandproper.com.au). I can't thank you enough for the amazing graphics in the book.

To my loving family. I wouldn't be here without my mum (my rock) and my dad. And one of the joys of modern-day living is being able to extend and blend your family, so I need to include Fred (you may be gone but your love and support is not forgotten) and Billie. I am so lucky to have not 1 but 2 phenomenal sisters: Vanessa and Laura I couldn't imagine life without either of you. Thank you for being there for me.

To my greatest asset, my daughter Emily. I'm actually grateful it just ended up being just the 2 of us. Being your mum has changed me in unbelievable ways. The strength and resilience that comes from solo parenting has made me, me. I love you more than you will ever know. I also need to thank you for allowing me time out to write, dream and grow. I can't imagine who I would have been if you didn't join me on this journey of life. And to the many people I have met because of this, Estelle Hughes, you came into my life to help with Emily as a newborn, who would have known you would stay forever and be my biggest spiritual guide. And to all my family, friends, and neighbours who have helped me survive so far. It takes a village to raise a child and I couldn't have done without everyone who pitched in along the way.

To Pat Flynn from Power Up Podcast, I have been talking about having a podcast for at least 5 years but never had the technical skills to get it up and running until I found you.

And to James Wedmore from Business By Design for turning the idea of a community into the Online Retreat. Again, this was an idle idea until you showed up and gave me the bite-sized steps to turn my dreams into a reality.

To Susan Dean, Natalie Deane and the Dean Publishing family for believing in my book.

Thank you.

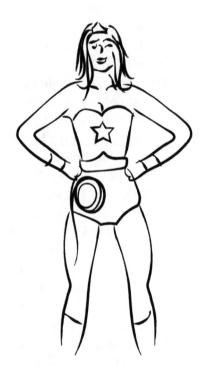

about the author

JENNIFER HARRINGTON N.D.
BACHELOR HEALTH SCIENCE
(NATUROPATHY)

Jennifer's interest in natural therapies started when she was diagnosed with polycystic ovary syndrome (PCOS) in her early twenties and was told she may struggle to have children. Initially she tried the oral contraceptive pill as prescribed by her doctor, but this didn't last long. The pain, mood swings and other side effects were unbearable; the stabbing sensation in her ovaries alone could drop her to the ground. Jennifer then tried naturopathy. Over time, her pain stopped, her cycles regulated and her fertility returned; a healing so significant she never looked back. Leaving her career in television,

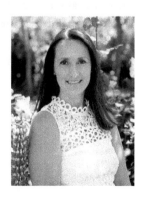

Jennifer retrained as a naturopath so she could help other women like herself.

Upon graduating, she moved to Thailand and started working at the famous Chiva Som International Health Resort. This afforded Jennifer an amazing experience and opportunity to rub shoulders with the best minds in industry, both from a traditional and modern medicine perspective.

Jennifer's love of retreats started here. She was inspired by the rapid transformation people could make outside of the distractions of their home environment; observing people leave the resort different to when they arrived. Recognising that healing and benefits could be fast-tracked, where months of work could be reduced to days, made a huge impression on Jennifer.

Jennifer returned to Sydney in 2005 to become a mum. She is eternally grateful she found naturopathy and was able to have a child after all.

After working in various Sydney based clinics and corporate health businesses, Jennifer decided it was time to open her own clinic in 2010. After advertising as a hormone specialist, she found she had more menopausal clients than fertility clients. The fast transformations that her menopausal clients were making made her rethink her work and she started Menopause Natural Solutions in 2014. As the years passed, she sold her brick-and-mortar clinic to free up time to dedicate herself to researching and creating a better way to help more perimenopausal and menopausal women. This book is an accumulation of five years of research, that has been tried and tested.

Today Jennifer lives in a beachside suburb of Sydney with her daughter Emily, their dog Missy and two guinea pigs. She enjoys being out in nature, travelling, socialising and continually learning.

testimonials

"What a fabulous resource. Jen has put together a wealth of information about how to negotiate the 'adventure' of menopause. She gives so many pearls of wisdom – about how to combat what many of us think of as "normal" suffering through this age-old rite of passage.

Jen is entertaining in her delivery of anecdotes and stories and the information and advice she shares is easy to understand and pleasantly informative. I'd recommend all women approaching menopause, anyone concerned about this next chapter in their lives or someone in the throes of this NORMAL stage of womanhood to definitely explore Jen's book.

You'll be entertained, empowered and quietly excited as she shows you how to make this transition gracefully. THANK YOU Jen for putting together a great resource in such an entertaining fashion. I've already ordered my ten copies to share with friends, family and patients. I want to help empower them to be warrior queens in menopause!"

Dr Sonya Floreani-Doherty
Chiropractor

"Jennifer Harrington has written a much needed book to help empower menopausal women to improved Health and Wellness.

There is a large void in the healthcare model with respect to treating the Real causes of disease and disability.

If we think of the health continuum as a process....from Optimal Health to Dysfunctional Health to Disease Health... then we quickly realise that disease just doesn't happen overnight, but that it's a gradual declining process over time. Often with no symptoms until the later stages!

It should therefore make sense to look back along each person's lifestyle timeline and implement a health care strategy to address the Why of your current health!?

There is a paradigm in natural health that says 'the body is self healing and self regulating '....so the goal of the Natural Therapist is to provide at an individual patient by patient level the strategies to promote healing healing by their own body. This is the basis of Natural Medicine! This process is supported by well considered and appropriate natural therapies such as naturopathy, chiropractic, and acupuncture.

This Natural Medicine approach can and should be used throughout each person's health journey as the cornerstone of support....even if the need for more radical Disease interventions is warranted.

Jennifer has a wealth of experience in the management of menopausal issues, and has kindly and generously shared her expertise in this book."

Dr Wayne Gard
Chiropractor. Naturopath. Acupuncturist

references

Menopause suffering is not about your hormones

https://www.reuters.com/article/us-health-menopause-perceptions/culture-may-influence-how-women-experience-menopause-idUSKBN0OL1XH20150605

Why western women suffer

Flint M. *The menopause: reward or punishment?* Psychosomatics. 1975.

Lock, Margaret. *Encounters with Aging: Mythologies of Menopause in Japan and North America.* Berkeley: University of California Press, 1993.=

Stefanopoulou, Shah, Shah, Gupta, Sturdee, and Hunter. *An International Menopause Society study of climate, altitude, temperature (IMS-CAT) and vasomotor symptoms in urban Indian regions.* Climacteric. 2014 Aug. Epub 2013 Nov 7.

https://www.swanstudy.org

https://www.ncbi.nlm.nih.gov/pmc/articles/PMC3613855/ – Pagan "Croning" ritual

https://en.wikipedia.org/wiki/Hag

What's happening on why

https://en.wikipedia.org/wiki/Estrogen_receptor#Distribution

https://news.wsu.edu/2017/05/03/toxic-effects-mercury-exposure-persists-multiple-generations-study-suggests/

https://www.fxmedicine.com.au/content/chronic-stress-cortisol-resistance-immunity

https://www.ewg.org/news/videos/10-americans

https://www.holisticprimarycare.net/latest-articles/1981-the-estrobolome-how-microbes-affect-estrogen-metabolism-cancer-risk.html

Nutritious food

https://responsibletechnology.org/gmo-education/gmos-in-food

https://www.biosolids.com.au/info/what-are-biosolids

https://www.ewg.org/foodnews/dirty-dozen.php

https://byronbaycoffeeco.com.au/mycotoxin-free-coffee

Dr Jason Fung "The Obesity Code"

Vitamins and minerals

https://ods.od.nih.gov/ – all vitamins

https://www.xcode.life/23andme-raw-data/beta-carotene-conversion-vitamin-a

https://www.drstevenlin.com/vitamin-k2-benefits

https://www.drugs.com/drug_interactions.html

https://www.ncbi.nlm.nih.gov/pubmed/16930085

https://www.drugs.com/drug-interactions/copper-gluconate,copper-index.html

http://pennstatehershey.adam.com/content.aspx?productId=107&pid=33&gid=000968

http://pennstatehershey.adam.com/content.aspx?productId=107&pid=33&gid=000344

https://lpi.oregonstate.edu/mic/minerals/manganese

Testing

EBV and menopause – Medical Medium Book by Anthony William

Non-toxic environment
References

Book: *Healthy home, healthy family* by Nicole Bijlmsa

Book: *Low Tox Life* by Alexx Stuart

Documentary: What's with wheat

https://mercola.com

https://www.survivingmold.com

Contribution

https://www.sciencedirect.com/science/article/pii/S1090513816300721

https://www.handsgroup.org.au

Exercise and other lifestyle factors
Sleep Research

https://www.ncbi.nlm.nih.gov/pubmed/26192072

https://www.ncbi.nlm.nih.gov/pubmed/26000551

https://www.ncbi.nlm.nih.gov/pubmed/29765930

https://www.ncbi.nlm.nih.gov/pubmed/24199972

Smoking

https://www.ncbi.nlm.nih.gov/pmc/articles/PMC4542296

https://www.pennmedicine.org/news/news-releases/2014/february/penn-medicine-study-reveals-ge

https://www.nature.com/articles/bjc2014132

https://www.icanquit.com.au/reasons-to-quit/smoking-and-your-health/health-dangers-of-smoking

https://www.ncbi.nlm.nih.gov/pmc/articles/PMC3530709

Love your Liver and detox

https://www.sciencedirect.com/science/article/pii/S0891552005701276

https://en.wikipedia.org/wiki/Viral_hepatitis

Specific problems
Hot flushes
https://www.ncbi.nlm.nih.gov/pubmed/11063896

https://sanescohealth.com/mechanism-of-hot-flashes

https://en.wikipedia.org/wiki/Norepinephrine

Sexual Health
https://www.ncbi.nlm.nih.gov/pubmed/18374688

Sexy brain by Dr Devaki Lindsey Berkson

DrNorthrup.com

https://www.youtube.com/user/drruth

https://www.youtube.com/watch?v=jf5_ZJlQqrY

Breast
Pinkhope.org.au

Breast cancer network australia

Bones
https://www.atsdr.cdc.gov/csem/csem.asp?csem=34&po=9

https://en.wikipedia.org/wiki/Hyperparathyroidism

Joint
https://www.ncbi.nlm.nih.gov/pmc/articles/PMC4226038

https://www.ncbi.nlm.nih.gov/pmc/articles/PMC2787275

Nerve health
https://www.mayoclinic.org/diseases-conditions/peripheral-neuropathy/care-at-mayo-clinic/mac-20352071

https://www.ncbi.nlm.nih.gov/pmc/articles/PMC5296423

https://ndnr.com/pain-medicine/ascending-progressive-polyneuropathy-treatment/

https://www.naturalmedicinejournal.com/journal/2010-08/therapeutic-effects-acetyl-l-carnitine-peripheral-neuropathy-review-literature

https://www.ncbi.nlm.nih.gov/pmc/articles/PMC5172536

Digestion
https://ubiome.com/clinical/smartgut

https://www.fxmedicine.com.au/content/stewed-healing-apples-and-immune-cofactors

Cognition
https://www.littlebrown.com/titles/jean-carper/100-simple-things-you-can-do-to-prevent-alzheimers-and-age-related-memory-loss/9780316121606

Urinary system
https://urogyn.coloradowomenshealth.com/patients/library/menopause-urinary-symptoms

https://www.mayoclinic.org/diseases-conditions/urinary-incontinence/diagnosis-treatment/drc-20352814

Headaches
https://www.ncbi.nlm.nih.gov/pmc/articles/PMC4117050

https://www.ncbi.nlm.nih.gov/pmc/articles/PMC3311830

Thyroid
https://www.ncbi.nlm.nih.gov/pubmed/27833448

https://www.ncbi.nlm.nih.gov/pmc/articles/PMC6166548

Skin
https://www.mdedge.com/cutis/article/106506/aesthetic-dermatology/skin-disorders-during-menopause

http://www.dermalinstitute.com/au/library/12_article_How_Does_Menopause_Affect_the_Skin_.html

Immune
https://www.ncbi.nlm.nih.gov/pmc/articles/PMC3954964

Headspace

https://www.health.harvard.edu/newsletter_article/generalized-anxiety-disorder

https://www.ncbi.nlm.nih.gov/pmc/articles/PMC4393509/

https://universityhealthnews.com/daily/depression/best-probiotics-for-mood-enhancing-the-gut-brain-connection-with-psychobiotics

https://www.ncbi.nlm.nih.gov/pubmed/19150053

http://shefayekhatam.ir/browse.php?a_id=1195&sid=1&slc_lang=en

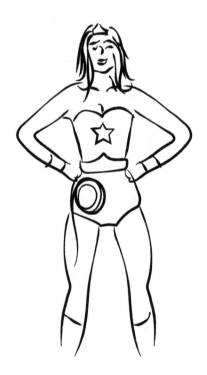

index

L

Libido 127, 130, 182, 201

Liver 15–17, 32, 35, 86, 109–112, 162, 175

L-lysine 154, 161, 196

M

MARCoNS 88

Meditation 104, 106, 119, 127, 154, 203, 204, 208

Menstruation 86, 125, 192

Migraine 68, 150, 170–174

Minerals

    Calcium 56, 58–60, 68, 69, 79, 80, 111, 140–141, 145, 164, 196

    Chromium 61, 178, 181

    Copper 62–63, 73, 82, 85, 86, 162, 180

    Iodine 12, 64–65, 87, 138, 184

    Iron 43, 44, 51, 59, 62, 66–67, 71, 72, 83, 86, 126, 146, 148, 153, 158, 162, 164, 180, 190

    Magnesium 12, 58, 59, 64, 68–70, 72, 75, 80, 106, 120, 121, 130, 141, 145, 147, 154, 164, 170, 173, 174, 181, 184, 196, 204, 205

    Manganese 71–72, 141, 153, 185, 196

    Molybdenum 73–74

    Potassium 64, 65, 68, 75–76, 80, 83, 141, 145, 164

    Selenium 64, 77–78, 154, 177, 184, 196

    Silica 79, 142, 190

    Sodium 64, 73, 75, 80–81, 145, 164

    Zinc 12, 45, 59, 63, 82–83, 86, 92, 142, 148, 152, 161, 170, 177, 184, 187, 190, 196

Mould 32, 38, 88, 94, 138, 155, 171, 174

N

N Acetyl Cysteine 154, 174, 190

Nails 79, 182

Neurotransmitters 33, 51, 103, 149, 158, 200

Night Sweat 15, 18, 117, 130–131, 202, 205

O

Omega 3 35, 129

Organic Food 29–30, 93, 111

Orgasm 132, 134, 135, 205

Osteoporosis 3, 36, 59, 60, 71, 79, 85, 87, 105, 139, 141, 143

Oxytocin 132

P

Pain 41, 52, 63, 64, 66, 69, 85, 86, 87, 94, 104, 111, 116, 120,

Printed in the USA
CPSIA information can be obtained
at www.ICGtesting.com
LVHW021256221123
764648LV00010B/228